A Public Health Strategy for Living, Aging, and Dying in Solidarity

With more people living longer lives, there is increased importance in the health care industry on improving services and supports for older persons. This comprehensive book gives an expert overview of the topics and challenges, along with imperative ethical and legal frameworks.

A Public Health Strategy for Living, Aging, and Dying in Solidarity also details existing programs and benefits in relation to a realistic portrayal of population needs. Other important issues are covered such as long-term care, palliative care and hospice, other vulnerable populations, elder abuse, public–private collaboration, evidence-based policy making, and much more.

Mary Beth Quaranta Morrissey is a Fellow at Fordham University's Global Healthcare Innovation Management Center and a health care attorney and aging and health researcher.

Melissa Lang is the Chief Executive Officer at Gilda's Club Westchester.

Barney Newman is Medical Director Emeritus for the WESTMED Medical Group, where he also served as the Chief Medical Officer.

Best Practices for Public Health

https:www.crcpress.com/Best-Practices-for-Public-Health/book-series/BPPH

Edited by Herman Koren, Indiana State University, USA

This series of books offers students, academics and practitioners invaluable practical guides. It adopts a global perspective and aims to drive practical action in an increasingly globalized world.

Best Practices for Environmental Health
Environmental Pollution, Protection, Quality and Sustainability
Herman Koren

A Public Health Strategy for Living, Aging, and Dying in Solidarity
Designing Elder-Centered and Palliative Systems of Care, Environments, Services, and Supports
Mary Beth Quaranta Morrissey, Melissa Lang, Barney Newman

A Public Health Strategy for Living, Aging, and Dying in Solidarity

Designing elder-centered
and palliative systems of care,
environments, services, and supports

**Mary Beth Quaranta Morrissey,
Melissa Lang, and Barney Newman**

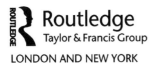

Routledge
Taylor & Francis Group

LONDON AND NEW YORK

First published 2019
by Routledge

2 Park Square, Milton Park, Abingdon, Oxfordshire OX14 4RN
52 Vanderbilt Avenue, New York, NY 10017

Routledge is an imprint of the Taylor & Francis Group, an informa business

First issued in paperback 2019

Library of Congress Cataloging-in-Publication Data

Names: Morrissey, Mary Beth Quaranta, author. | Lang,
Melissa (Melissa Mary), author. | Newman, Barney,
author.
Title: A public health strategy for living, aging, and dying
in solidarity : designing elder-centered and palliative
systems of care, environments, services, and supports /
Mary Beth Morrissey, Melissa Lang, Barney Newman.
Description: Abingdon, Oxon ; New York, NY : Routledge,
2018. | Includes bibliographical references and index.
Identifiers: LCCN 2018005541| ISBN 9781498761345
(hardback) | ISBN 9781315367606 (ebook)
Subjects: | MESH: Health Services for the Aged--
organization & administration | Palliative Care | Long-
Term Care | Patient-Centered Care | United States
Classification: LCC RC952.5 | NLM WT 31 | DDC
618.97029--dc23
LC record available at https://lccn.loc.gov/2018005541

ISBN: 978-1-4987-6134-5 (hbk)
ISBN: 978-1-367-45748-8 (pbk)

To Lawrence O. Gostin and his Dad, Joseph Gostin

Contents

Foreword

It's all there in the title of *A Public Health Strategy for Living, Aging and Dying in Solidarity*. Rarely does a book pose such key challenges and predicaments for society as this important work by three pioneers in academia and social service, public health and medical care. Their informative and action-oriented chapters call upon the reader to grasp and reflect on three things, above all.

First, the meaning of *aging*. Demographic trends and the experience of historically unprecedented life-spans for large numbers of people will reshape institutions and expectations. They will tax our human and financial resources and society's capability to meet special needs. They will pose philosophical and ethical questions that we are, at the moment, unprepared to answer.

Next, the meaning of living and aging *well*. In the context of growing old, and especially in the existential confrontation with the vagaries of extreme old age, what is the best way to honor the human rights and core values that inform the meaning of living well? What does it mean to flourish—to continue to enjoy the rights of life, liberty, and the pursuit of happiness—as one lives with progressive, chronic illness, frailty, or dementia?

In addition, when it comes to dying well, how can we fulfill the promise of respect for individual rights, relief of suffering, and providing care for meaningful dignity to the very end? How can we further improve decision making near the end of life, and how can be provide better access to palliative care and hospice services?

Finally, the prospect of a *public health strategy*. To view something as a matter of public health is to think in terms of populations of people, rather than in terms of providing service to one person at a time. Moreover, to comprehend trends such as aging, or services such as long-term care or palliative care, from a public health perspective is to focus on patterns of human behavior and on the social and natural environment within which behavior related to health or illness takes place. A public health perspective is "ecological" in that it examines the relationships and interactions between groups and individuals socially and the natural environmental factors that influence their health.

The action strategy that flows from such a relational or ecological perspective strives to bring about improvement in the health and well-being of populations and individuals by looking at the big picture of institutional, cultural, and structural power that influences the choices and life-styles that individuals make.

A Public Health Strategy for Living, Aging and Dying in Solidarity gives welcome and special attention to suffering in old age and to palliative care as a public health issue. But many other aspects of aging well lend themselves to a public health approach, as well, and indeed are related to suffering. Poor diet is an example.

A physician counseling an individual patient might ask why the person eats so much sugary and fatty foods and advise against doing that. A public health perspective would ask why more healthy food choices are neither available nor affordable in poor neighborhoods where this patient may live. Public health would ask how diet related health factors could be improved by changes in the agricultural and food processing system and by addressing economic inequality and environmental justice in access to healthy food choices. For the growing number of persons over age 85 who are living with frailty, public health related programs that change institutional structures and provide personal empowerment, like Meals-on-Wheels, play a vital role in aging well.

In sum, aging can be viewed from a public health and systemic perspective as well as a biographical life course and clinical one. To take a public health perspective is to be concerned with population health and aging, based on research in demographics and epidemiology, seeking patterns in large scale health and function. Moreover, to take a public health perspective is to be especially attentive to institutional structure and resource access—which are largely artifacts of public policy—as they affect the capabilities of individuals, families, and groups to flourish as they grow old.

Successful or healthy aging is a challenge for a society as a whole, not simply something that individuals and families should have to cope with on their own. An aging society is defined as one in which there are more individuals over 65 than under 15. To make a successful adaptation or transition to an aging society is a historically unusual, indeed unprecedented, test that we are facing now. With what ethical vision, what political will, and what institutional organization of public policy and social provision will America be able to pass that test?

Mary Beth Morrissey, and co-authors Melissa Lang, and Barney Newman, exemplify the strength and promise of interdisciplinary scholarship and analysis. Together they bring to this topic and book wide experience and expertise in the fields of medicine, law, social work, counseling, health policy, palliative care and biomedical ethics. If the test of our society's successful adaptation to aging can be passed, these thinkers provide a valuable tutorial.

The American health care system continues to roil politically over how to reform private health insurance markets and how to incentivize health care providers to contain costs and provide appropriate and timely medical care to their communities. Amid all this, however, there is essentially no health insurance for long-term care, with the exception of a governmental means-tested program designed originally to provide primary and preventive services to those with very low income and assets. No elder-centered system of care is possible under these conditions. The knowledge and creativity are there to achieve such a system. What is lacking is a political system capable of acting and a leadership willing to act. Also lacking, unfortunately, is a sufficient sense of intergenerational solidarity in our culture to believe that most people can live well in the final chapters of a long life. Yet, they can, and it is morally important that they be supported in doing so. An important step in the direction of rebuilding such solidarity is to take to heart the ecological and relational framework presented in this book.

Bruce Jennings is Adjunct Associate Professor at the Vanderbilt University School of Medicine and Senior Advisor at The Hastings Center.

Bruce Jennings

Introduction

The twenty-first century has ushered in a new era of elder care centered on understanding the first-person perspectives of older persons and their suffering in the ecological contexts of community, culture, and society. This person-centered approach recognizes older persons' lived experiences of suffering in aging, as well as their opportunities for resilience, meaning-making, and comfort in all domains of living and dying. This book's focus, a public health strategy for living, aging, and dying in solidarity in America, examines the meanings of aging and dying, as well as growing old across the lifespan, and challenges more conventional paradigms of successful aging. It provides a blueprint for improving the "quality of life and "quality of dying" for older Americans through radical change in social policy and social structures. The key pillar of such a public health strategy is population-level policy—both policy development and policy implementation, and translation of policy and its theoretical underpinnings into evidence-based model programs and effective practices to improve elder-centered care and enhance opportunities for elder flourishing, citizenship, and engagement with community. Policy centered on the goals of improving equitable access to education across the lifespan, as well as strengthening aging and health care workforce education and training, exemplifies a public health policy intervention capable of making a marked impact on elder health and well being over the next decades. Building societal conditions that make it possible for older persons to strive toward realizing their capacities and fulfilling their agency, even through their last days, must be a policy priority.

As we approach the end of the second decade of this century, we must take stock of the state of older adult health and well being, from multiple perspectives. In this book, we chart what the next decades will look like—for the older person and citizen, for family and professional caregivers, and for the diverse communities, cultures, and ecologies across the nation and globe. Scholars, planners, researchers, and professionals from a range of disciplines have committed themselves to this task of examining the important subject of aging through the lens of public health and public health policy–based responses to aging.

The goals of the present book are interdisciplinary. The authors' contributions reflect expertise across a number of disciplines—public health, gerontology, law, policy, psychology, social work, medicine, and ethics. The prominent focus on the social and, more specifically, the social-ecological perspective, aligns with directions in aging and health policy today, which are oriented toward more seamless elder- and family-centered systems of care and the increasing integration of medical and social services. In drawing on ecological and social theory to inform and guide understanding of complex problems of older adults, we seek to foster an interdisciplinary balance in the aging and public health fields and to place older adults and their social problems in the context of their environments and a global world. We believe our interdisciplinary approach helps lay a foundation for the central, unifying themes that emerge from the breadth of theoretical and practical orientations. Among these themes are:

- The priority of the older person and elder-centered ethics in the design and provision of care and the allocation of scarce resources.
- Integration of a public health strategy in the formulation of policy and the design of geriatric health and palliative systems of care and environments for aging comfortably, informed and guided by theoretical frameworks.
- The translation of theory into evidence-based model programs and effective practices.
- Advancing social ecological approaches to governance to modify the social and economic determinants of elder health and well being.

Throughout the book, aging people and populations will be placed in the context of the social systems, communities, and environments in which they are functionally embedded.

The book is organized into four parts:

- Part One: The Crisis of Suffering for Older Americans
- Part Two: Paradigm Shifts in Delivery Systems and Financing
- Part Three: Challenges in Policy Implementation: Examples from the Field
- Part Four: Setting the Stage for Transforming Elder Care

In each of these sections, we examine the role of theory and evidence, as well as law and regulation, in shaping the life-world of older persons as the beneficiaries of aging and health policy. We also identify policy gaps and failures, as well as successes. Reflecting the authors' different backgrounds and areas of expertise, the sections move from meta-theoretical perspectives and public health policy considerations to practical strategies for addressing problems in the design and implementation of delivery systems along with financing, programs, and best practices. Special emphasis in this book is given to the role of palliative care in transforming systems of elder care and its implications for the related professions. The book concludes with recommendations for policy reform that we believe may have the biggest impact on public health and on health and well being outcomes for older persons. In that category, we highlight the priority of education, and investments in education, for people across their entire lifespan as yielding the richest benefits for society as a whole.

In all of this, we do wish to be fully transparent with our readers in communicating that this book provides no clinical information or guidance about older adults' medical care or mental health needs. Our principal focus is policy and the design of aging, health, and public health systems.

Before proceeding, we would like to make some general comments about the writing style, voice, and terminology. One implication of integrating these different authors and levels of analysis is that the writing shifts considerably between different chapters to reflect the book's dual function, which is on the one hand theoretical and philosophical, and on the other hand concrete and practical. Chapters 1, 2, 7, and 8, reflecting Mary Beth Quaranta Morrissey's background in public health law and policy, ethics, and theoretical psychology, draw upon a rich set of theoretical resources offered by phenomenology and certain schools of ethics, which have not traditionally been systematically applied to the arenas of gerontology and palliative care. Phenomenology is a rigorous scientific method utilized in the study of consciousness and lived experience, such as consciousness of suffering. Phenomenological studies of suffering among older adults help to illuminate the meanings of suffering through opening the field of experience to a critical understanding of the person and personhood. This ethically rooted understanding informs the formulation of policy and the social justice imperatives of policy. The authors identify palliative care, which may be generally described as specialized medical care or socially directed supportive care that aims to relieve pain and suffering, as a burgeoning area of policy development that will heavily influence care for older adults generally. The philosophical bent of these chapters can make for a tough read, but is necessary to provide a proper foundation for the book's larger vision. The other chapters, reflecting Barney Newman's and Melissa Lang's backgrounds in medicine and public health, respectively, engage with fundamental policy and practice considerations that complement, and ultimately follow from, such theory. In addition, given that aging and the design of palliative systems of care for all aging persons as a *public health* (not just medical) issue are often overshadowed in the national conversation, a concerted effort is made to familiarize the reader with the historical background and current landscape of this field. Accordingly, these chapters and introductory sections are highly fact-based and methodical, anchored in the structural and legal realities of public policy, bureaucracy, and system management; they show where the "rubber meets the road" in practical terms. The book's status as both a theoretical *and* applied enterprise lends itself well, we feel, to a subject matter that is arguably just as relevant to ethics and lived experience as it is to the urgencies of policy implementation, costs, and demographic considerations.

While the book's broad focus encompasses both global and national policy, sections of certain chapters bear a distinct "New York" voice. In many instances, case studies and examples of models of care are New York–based. However, the integration of global, national, and local perspectives balances the authors' New York identities.

We offer one final note here about our use of terminology throughout the book. Generally, we have favored the term "older person" rather than "elder" to describe a person who is aging or has reached her or his later years. We believe that this term is the least stigmatizing of the options available. Such a distinction speaks, once again, to our deeply held belief that terminology matters a great deal when it comes to the kind of paradigm shift in aging and public health care that we envision. However, at points in the book, we may use the term "elder" as a noun or adjective, such as "elder care" or "elder-centered care," mainly to avoid awkward language constructions. At all times, it is our intent to show the highest respect and consideration for all older persons.

The authors would like to thank Lawrence O. Gostin, Bruce Jennings, Frederick J. Wertz, and Michael Barber for their contributions to the book's scholarship.

The authors would also like to acknowledge the following individuals who provided generous assistance and support in the editing of the manuscript: Allison Peltzman, Christopher Schuck, and Madeleine Haig.

Part One

The crisis of suffering for older Americans

1   Social ecology of aging
Critical theoretical perspectives in aging and public health policy for the twenty-first century

I. Introduction

As we approach the end of the second decade of the twenty-first century amidst relative chaos in the national policy arena, policy makers are positioned to seize upon a rare horizon of opportunity to alter the trajectory of suffering that characterizes growing old in America. More specifically, policy makers can mitigate elder suffering associated with both societal conditions and the burdens of individual illness and functional limitations, and they can afford elders the chance to live and age comfortably, *and* to die in solidarity. By living, aging, and dying in solidarity, we mean to suggest Aristotelian notions of flourishing that implicate meanings of community and subjective and inter-subjective well being or *eudaimonia* (Drummond, 2002; Steptoe, Deaton, & Stone, 2015), but we expand upon those notions of well being by including within their purview meanings of "palliative," such as dwelling in the palliative embrace of supportive communities. An Aristotelian sense of well being is related to the intentionalities, teleological and vocational life goals, and purposes of a moral agent, and the fulfillment of intentionalities in light of such individual goals, as well as the goods of moral agency itself as philosopher John Drummond (2002, 2008) has explicated.

Now more than any other time, policy makers and policy advocates—together with the older adult stakeholders on whose behalf they commit themselves—must converge on the vortex in the political economy of the early twenty-first century to forge coalitions, mount active resistance to regressive policy, and lead change processes that will directly impact and nullify conditions of oppression and suffering that burden older Americans and interfere with their attainment of life goals. We call upon such policy makers, advocates, and coalitions, including older adults themselves in diverse roles, to work collaboratively as agents for change, building environments that make conditions possible for palliation of elder suffering, elder flourishing, resilience in the midst of suffering, and the fostering of elders' deep relational connection with meaningful others and their community. In this chapter, we focus on understanding the manifold environmental layers that shape the experience of suffering and growing old in America, including the complexity of social systems and the recalcitrance and inhospitability of the aging and public health sectors themselves—what we describe as the *social ecology of aging*. Drawing on the history of various movements in aging and person-centered care, including the tensions around the goals of such movements, we reframe the goals of living, aging, and dying, as comfortably and palliatively as reasonably possible, in fundamentally social terms. In light of the main sociopolitical and economic drivers of aging and health policy, we propose an elder-centered care approach that responds to the social suffering of older persons and addresses inequities in accessing essential health and social services, supports, and care.

The goals of an elder-centered care frame are multiple:

- To define the social problem of suffering for all older persons, especially vulnerable, frail and seriously ill older persons.
- To identify structural and systems barriers to older persons' pursuit of life goals, flourishing, and comfort.
- To raise awareness of elder needs and rights.
- To inform and guide policy planning and the development of model programs and effective practices.
- To craft public health and global public health agendas designed to change the current paradigm to one more capable of meeting the needs of older people in their social, cultural, and community contexts.

Such a paradigm shift involves changing the conditions of older adults' embedded environments, modifying social and economic determinants of health, and, according to public health law scholar Lawrence O. Gostin (2014), making comprehensive health goods, services, and facilities *available, accessible, affordable, and acceptable*, both ethically and culturally. The right to health requires nothing less.

This chapter is organized into four main sections:

- Defining the social problem of elder suffering in the context of the environmental landscape.
- Describing the social ecology of aging and its principal ecosystems.
- Addressing the shift to elder-centered care.
- Explicating an elder-centered public health strategy for improving elder health and well being.

II.   Framing the social problem of elder suffering: Social ecological and environmental contexts

A *sine qua non* of policy development in aging and health is understanding the nature of the principal social problem that drives aging and health policy making: the problem of suffering. In this chapter, we describe the magnitude of the problem and its critical dimensions as part of an overview of the larger social ecological and environmental landscape, as well as argue for a firm and settled commitment to change policy that has a detrimental impact on older adult beneficiaries. The types of factors shaping the landscape of global suffering for Americans as they age into their later years include individual-level variables; variables at the sociopolitical, economic, and cultural level; and factors that have both micro- and macrosystem implications and consequences. For example, chronic conditions, functional limitations, and disability burdens have a direct impact on elders' personal health status, but also have important systems implications. A goal of this chapter is to explicate the complex entanglements and relationships of experiences and outcomes for the older person as an individual in relation to the larger systems in which they are embedded. In addition to personal health characteristics, among the mix of factors we consider and discuss in this chapter are sociopolitical movements; ecology of policy; demographic trends; caregiving resources and risks of elder abuse; social and economic determinants of health and inequities in access to care; inadequacy of aging, health, and social systems, including community-based services and supports; workforce gaps; a rapidly changing climate ecology and concomitant risks of displacement and homelessness; and inadequate understanding, assessment and measurement of suffering. These multidimensional factors are described and discussed more fully below.

III. Social ecology of aging and its ecosystems: Interaction of macro- and microsystems

Essential to the aging and public health focus of this book is describing *a social ecology of aging* and its *ecosystems*. The social ecological perspective on elder human development, drawn on throughout the book and explicated in this chapter, helps to make sense of the range of lived experiences of growing old—the multiple faces of suffering, including vulnerability, frailty, limitation, and dependency, as well as agency, growth, flourishing, and relational connection. The book's chapters are organized around key questions to help unpack the critical components of the ecology of aging in its breadth, depth, and complexity:

• Who comprises the older adult population of interest and the stakeholders in elders' families and communities that are the book's focus?
• What are the critical policies, programs, and benefits intended to serve older people?
• What delivery and financing systems for such policies and programs exist, and what kinds of delivery and financing systems are ideal?
• What innovations in approaches to care hold promise for transforming older persons' lives, health, and well being?

Encompassing multi-level systems theory, an interdisciplinary ecosystem framework has been adopted widely in work with older adults across all settings, although it remains under-developed and under-resourced. Adopting a social ecological, systems lens on aging and public health is based on the logic that it can help disentangle the social and economic structures in the larger environmental landscape in which older persons are situated, both to enhance understanding of the influence of these structures on their life-worlds and enable design of improved public health and care systems. The social ecological perspective fits well with a public health approach to aging as it takes account of factors such as elder access to clean water, food, housing, transportation, and health and supportive services that are shaping the aging experience and constrain and marginalize the power of the elderly person as individual to change her/his experience, environment, and health and well being outcomes. In this chapter, we recognize the reciprocal relationship between health and human rights (Gostin, 2014) and what that relationship means in terms of access to care.

A.   *Social ecological perspective on human development*

The social ecological perspective on human development is well established in interdisciplinary fields of aging and public health (Bronfenbrenner, 1979; Garbarino, 1999; Cox, 2005, 2007; Meyer, 1983; Pincus & Minahan, 1973; Wakefield, 1996). Going back several decades, Urie Bronfenbrenner (1979) developed a conceptual framework of a person situated in her or his environment based upon how the person perceives and experiences that environment. Bronfenbrenner's framework influenced many other thinkers including his former student, James Garbarino. Citing Edmund Husserl, the founder of phenomenology, psychologist Kurt Lewin, and others, Bronfenbrenner (1979) describes the ecological view as phenomenological in nature in its attention to perception and lived experience, and he gives it primacy over the physical and objective environment in understanding human behavior. Ecological perspectives have descriptive power, rather than predictive or explanatory applications, and are rooted in approaches to social problems that encompass a dual focus on the individual and the society (Meyer, 1983; Mullaly, 2007; Wakefield, 1996). Consistent with the strengths perspective of social work, the social ecological orientation adopts a strengths-based perspective toward human development, focusing on a person's assets and resilience in overcoming risks (Saleebey, 2006). Carol Meyer's (1983) seminal work in the social work field established the ecosystems perspective as necessary in social work, and it underscored the non-linear relationship and interaction between the person and the environment, including its systems and sub-systems (Wakefield, 1996). Critical perspectives on the political economy of aging also employ micro-, meso-, and macro-level analysis to examine social and structural influences on the problems of older adults and other vulnerable populations, such as women, who have historically been marginalized in the society (Estes et al., 2001; Abramovitz, 2009).

Person- and elder-centered approaches to care offer the possibility of development across the lifespan, building on both personal and community assets. Garbarino's (1999) contributions to social ecology have focused on youth, but they have important implications for older adults and their development in later years. Drawing on Bronfenbrenner, Garbarino charts a developmental trajectory for youth that balances consideration of accumulation of risks and accumulation of opportunities, with an emphasis on understanding the trajectories of resilience, the potentialities for personal growth, and the limits to resilience in social context. Garbarino (1999) identifies spirituality—the belief in something larger than oneself—as a *sine qua non* in this delicate balance. Garbarino's research suggests that youth who cannot make sense of the meaningfulness of their lives are at higher risk for violence than those who are spiritually centered. These findings have important implications for older persons, their life goals, meaning projects, and capacities for agency and resilience. While in its origins ecological systems theory focused on youth, it is now being used in work with many other populations including older adults with dementia and nursing home residents, and has implications for their health and well being and their lifespan trajectories (Blevins & Deason-Howell, 2002; Cox, 2005, 2007; Lepore, Miller, & Gozalo, 2011; Morgan & Brosi, 2007; Gonzalez Sanders & Fortinsky, 2012).

The idea of human development is well documented in psychology and the human sciences from Freud to Piaget, Erikson, and Winnicott (Guntrip, 1971). The important contribution of Bronfenbrenner (1979) and Garbarino (1999) to this literature is their focus on social context. They build on the work of previous thinkers in elaborating on the systems view to develop a complex structural mapping of the environment in which persons function and interact among themselves and with the inorganic environment (Lyman & Alvarez de Toledo, 2006). Applying ecological systems theory to older adults, we identify the various units or layers of the social ecological environment enveloping each older person:

- The older adult is embedded in an individually distinct microsystem through which the older adult experiences everyday life in direct contact with surrounding systems.
- The mesosystem comprises multiple interrelated organizational and social systems in which the older adult participates that also have a direct influence on the older adult.
- Finally, the macrosystem is constituted largely by societal norms; policies; cultural beliefs; various economic, political, and other structures; language; and ideologies that have a consistency across all the underlying systems and exert an influence on the older adult and other structures.

According to Compton, Galaway, and Cournoyer (2005), in addition to the above enumerated layers of the environment, another layer, the situational layer, applies to the individual's perceived environment stemming from one's immediate temporal and spatial experience. This book principally focuses on the interaction between the micro- and macro-environments, beginning with an analysis of macrosystems and structures.

The organismic systems viewpoint and the human development-specific strands of the social ecological model provide a rich tool for investigating older adults' lived experiences, especially experiences of suffering and decision making. Ecological models and perspectives have been cited extensively in the foundational gerontological literature and have helped in assessments of the functioning, care, and support needs of older adults (Cox, 2005, 2007; Jopp, Rott, & Oswald, 2008; Oswald, Jopp, Rott, & Wahl, 2011). For example, Lawton and Nahemow's (1973) development of the "environmental press" model in the 1970s made an early contribution to this body of work by describing the relationshp between a given setting and an individual's capacities to function optimally in that setting, and calling for interventions either to modify the setting as appropriate or address an older adult's functional capabilities when the ecological balance is disrupted (Cox, 2005; Oswald et al., 2011). Eco-maps have been useful in assessments, relationship-charting, supports, and resources for older adults, including older adults with dementia, and they help delineate the qualitative nature of ties and relationships (Cox, 2007; Gonzalez Sanders & Fortinsky, 2012). Such mapping aids professional service providers in both planning and practice with family members (Cox, 2007). Saleebey (2006), a pioneer of the ecological model, relied on the work of Bronfenbrenner, whom he includes among the developmental ecologists, to conceptualize a developmental infrastructure for supportive communities that draws on multiple realities and resources. Such an approach is useful to aging and health professionals working in nursing facility, institutional, and community-based settings with older persons whose communities and infrastructures have collapsed.

Eric J. Cassell (2004) recognized the significance of the ecological perspective in his writing on suffering, although he acknowledged its slow adoption in the field of medicine. Morrissey and Jennings's (2006) social ecology of health model in the area of relational end-of-life decision making synthesizes the systems viewpoint from biology and environmental science, and acknowledges the "complex nexus of social and cultural relations among human beings" in individuals' lived experiences of illness at the end of life (Morrissey & Jennings, 2006, p. 55). Blevins and Deason-Howell (2002) apply Bronfenbrenner's model to nursing home residents at the end of life in examining the interface of policy, practice, and research.

The ecosystems framework is not without critique. Limitations of the systems and ecological perspectives that have been identified include their failure to address conflict, to confront differentials in power, or to acknowledge historical factors and oppressive social structures (Mullaly, 2007). Others have critiqued the biologically oriented conceptualizations of environmental adaptation, which do not account for the power of relationship building and individual agency in environmental change processes (Guntrip, 1971).

In this book, we argue for an ecological and ecosystems perspective that moves beyond notions of adaptation and instead emphasizes stronger and deeper relational connections as essential underpinnings in working with older adults. A growing body of work in psychology supports and advances relational approaches to flourishing and well being (Fowers, Richardson, & Slife, 2017).

B. Ecosystems in the social ecology of aging

1. Macrosystem: Law, policy, structures, and barriers to accessing care

Law and policy play a major role in aging and public health. It might even be said that there is an ecology of policy impacting older adults that makes up one province of the larger social ecology of aging. (See Appendix B, Ecology of Policy: Description of Public Policy Making Process.) The macrosystem comprises government, the welfare state, other broad social and economic policies, societal and cultural norms, ideologies, beliefs and expectations, and consistent phenomena or processes across the other underlying systems within the macrosystem. In this book, we examine international legal frameworks and human rights conventions as well as U.S. laws and policies.

In Bronfenbrenner's exposition on elements of the macrosystem in his major work *Ecology of Human Development* (1979), he stresses that the environment and its constituent systems are involved in dynamic processes of multi-level change that have their own trajectories. In other words, the environment is not static. What this means practically for older persons is that they are affected by law, policy, and social processes across the different settings in which they are situated.

According to Bronfenbrenner (1979), developmental changes may not be evident until an older person moves from a primary setting that may have been maintaining a certain level of functioning to another setting that may demand the older person take initiative to find new sources of stimulation and support. This hypothesis suggests an ecological trajectory that can survive transitions to new settings and can act as an impetus and support for personal growth and change (Bronfenbrenner, 1979). This is an important concept for older persons, who are sometimes transferred into residential settings from the security and comfort of their own homes or transferred to other systems for care at points in their clinical course. The capacity of systems to undergo and accommodate change is relevant to questions of agency, self-efficacy, and resilience for older persons facing challenges with chronic and serious illness and at the end of life. Drawing on the work of the psychoanalysts and developmentalists, Guntrip (1971) argues, however, that social adaptation and survival do not adequately account for an individual's psychic realities, meaning in relationships, and agency.

Importantly, and as discussed more fully, the macrosystem can also significantly constrain human development, growth, and resilience. Gutheil and

Congress (2000) and Castro and Zautra (2016) have linked resilience to social contexts and social bonds, drawing on research that shows that the quality and strength of relational connections and social support play an important role in the ability to accommodate change and overcome risk in later life.

A.   SOCIOPOLITICAL MOVEMENTS AND PARADIGM SHIFTS

For over half a century, the aging experience in America has been dominated by concepts of "successful aging" (Flatt et al., 2013; Havighurst, 1961; Rowe, 2015; Rowe & Kahn, 1987, 1997, 1998; Rubinstein & de Medeiros, 2015), or alternate iterations, such as productive aging, aging well, or "active aging" (World Health Organization [WHO], 2002). The "successful aging" movement in gerontology, driven by notions of autonomy and independence, emphasizes action, change, personal responsibility, and control at the individual level—notions that according to Flatt and colleagues (2013) have been nearly universally accepted. These notions posit that the aging or older individual has the capacity to control and even direct the aging process through the exercise of personal autonomy, choice, and decision making. As a consequence of such control, people succeed to varying degrees in improving the quality of the aging experience and even altering own individual outcomes, such as physical and cognitive health (Flatt, Settersten, Ponsaran, & Fishman, 2013; Havighurst, 1961). Some view this philosophy as a product of a neoliberal political economy (Flatt, Settersten, Ponsaran, & Fishman, 2013; Rubinstein & de Medeiros, 2015), with its emphasis on individual action. While the "successful aging" movement has seen critiques, including contestations of the meanings of "successful aging" from the field of anti-aging medicine, which has sought to alter the biological process of aging (Flatt, Settersten, Ponsaran, & Fishman, 2013), and revisions to the movement's individual-focused goals by architects of the movement themselves (Rowe, 2015), the movement has flourished. Postmodern culture and political economy, dominated by market-based, neoliberal ideologies, view aging as a modifiable condition of the environment and glorify the consumer—including the aging or older adult consumer—as a type of decision maker. The construction of the identity of this consumer type rests on a near-platonic ideal of a consumer, attributed with rationality, non-relationality, and self-governance, who is making choices without social or economic constraint. In addition to incorporating the rational choice theory of economics, neoliberalism promotes a narrative of the individual as a self-contained, self-possessed, and independent actor divorced from historical, social, and cultural contexts (Sugarman, 2015, 2017). In this book, we pay attention to the older Americans who, although overlooked in the neoliberal worldview, make up the majority of the older population: those older adults who fall outside this narrative, who may have fewer years of education and fewer resources, and who, as a result, may not be in a position to age well without significant social and economic support.

The underpinnings of neoliberalism are deeply rooted in American history, society, and culture (Sugarman, 2015, 2017), founded upon the pillars of rugged individualism and market liberalism and capitalism (Jennings, 1999, 2016; Fowers, Richardson, & Slife, 2017). However, it's important to disentangle neoliberalism and its incentives from market liberalism, which can be traced back to the eighteenth century and the emergence of capitalism in the context of nation and empire-building (Mullaly, 2007). The hallmarks of market liberalism were commitment to free trade, including the freedom to sell labor and own land and capital, the right to have a voice in governance, separation between church and state, and secularization. The evolution of market liberalism through the nineteenth century gave rise to a new form of social liberalism in the early twentieth century in response to inequality and failures of government. Franklin Delano Roosevelt's New Deal policies and Lyndon Baines Johnson's Great Society programs were examples of this social ideological turn. At least one commentator (Chowkwanyun, 2018) has highlighted the contributions of Johnson's War on Poverty to strengthening the health care safety net through integrated health and social care and improved community governance models. According to Chowkwanyun (2018), this historical precedent has implications for today's movement to create a "culture of health" (p. 47).

The economic crisis of the 1970s during the Reagan era marked another significant milestone in the evolution of liberalism, hailing the form of liberalism now commonly called *neoliberalism.*

Although neoliberalism did not emerge prominently until the 1970s, it is characterized by certain hallmark features. Sugarman (2015) offers a comprehensive description of neoliberalism and these distinctive features:

> "Neoliberalism" marks the overthrow of Keynesian welfare state economics by the Chicago School of political economy in the closing decades of the 20th century (Harvey, 2005; Palley, 2005). Its key features are a radically free market in which competition is maximized, free trade achieved through economic deregulation, privatization of public assets, vastly diminished state responsibility over areas of social welfare, the corporatization of human services, and monetary and social policies congenial to corporations and disregardful of the consequences: poverty, rapid depletion of resources, irreparable damage to the biosphere, destruction of cultures, and erosion of liberal democratic institutions (Brown, 2003). However, the reach of neoliberalism is even more extensive. Neoliberalism is reformulating personhood, psychological life, moral and ethical responsibility, and what it means to have selfhood and identity.
>
> (Sugarman, 2015, pp. 103–104)

Distinguishing neoliberalism from classical or market liberalism in its structural privileging of entrepreneurial activity over and against mere participation in economic life, Sugarman (2015) makes a powerful connection between neoliberalism as a political philosophy and its threats to personhood. Building on Sugarman's conceptualization of neoliberalism, we elaborate further here on the differentiation of neoliberalism from earlier forms of market liberalism and capitalism by the globalization turn—namely, the triumph of capitalism as a global system and the parallel triumph of globalization over nationalism.

Exploring these same themes, Jennings (1999) weighs the influential role of liberalism—and the doctrine of "liberal neutrality"—as a political theory that seeks to limit the role of the state to that of a neutral intermediary. According to Jennings (2016), Enlightenment culture and liberalism gave rise to a market-based social contract of consumption and to its fruits—namely, what Jennings calls "a secularized world view" and the loss or "privatization of the transcendent" (p. 62).

Rooted in liberalism and liberal neutrality are commonly held beliefs about the rights and liberty interests of individuals protected by the U.S. Constitution and by its body of jurisprudence, as well as certain state constitutions and statutes. Americans hold sacred these beliefs about the primacy of the rights and liberty of individuals going back to the nation's earliest history, and still prioritize them today in their schema of values. They are also reflected in policy, including judicial rulings. In the context of health care decision making by older adults with serious illness or at the end of their lives, the 1990 U.S. Supreme Court decision in *Cruzan v. Director, Missouri Department of Health* (1990) that recognized the constitutional right to refuse treatment stands as a prime example of such policy. The U.S. Supreme Court decision in *Cruzan* (1990), reasoning from which was later incorporated by the Court in *Vacco v. Quill* (1997) and *Washington v. Glucksberg* (1997) holding that state bans on assistance in committing suicide do not violate the Fourteenth Amendment, recognized the constitutional right to refuse treatment as grounded in a fundamental liberty interest protected by the Due Process Clause of the Fourteenth Amendment.

A contemporary example of a shift from a position of liberal neutrality to neoliberal-driven interests in aging and health policy is the attempted move from the constitutional right to refuse treatment to arguments for a constitutional right to aid in dying, also known as physician assistance in dying. The proponents of aid in dying argue that the right to self-determination, which includes the right to refuse medical treatment and to control the course of one's treatment, also encompasses a right to choose aid in dying and to control the manner of dying as natural extensions of forgoing treatment. In these arguments, the competent adult who would seek to hasten her or his death through aid in dying is positioned as a type of entrepreneur who would be pursuing the project of liberty in designing her or his own death in solitary fashion, removed from all relation and social connections, and the larger community or social order. This portrait of the neoliberal actor divorced from social contexts who seeks to hasten her or his death, yet who remains embedded in a neoliberal culture and ecosystem that prioritizies return on investment and marginalizes persons whose disabilities or functional limitations threaten to diminish such return, calls to mind sociologist Émile Durkheim's (1897/1997) sociological treatises on suicide and solidarity. In these treatises, Durkheim (1897/1997) describes an inverse relationship between rates of suicide in a society and the degree of integration of that society and its social groups, and cites excessive individualism and disintegration of social bonds as manifestations of a less highly integrated society from which suicide springs. Durkheim's remarkable insights into social structures and their impact on human persons and personhood provide a meaningful context for a closer examination of the aid in dying movement and its social ideological underpinnings.

Recent commentary on the goals of the aid-in-dying movement and on particular bills, such as the New York Medical Aid in Dying Act (A.2383, S.3151), have highlighted the absence of any dialogue about social structures and equity, for example, such as access to education, in weighing the considerations involved in the crafting of a medical aid-in-dying right or benefit (Abbott, Glover, & Wynia, 2017; New York City Bar Association, 2017). While the constitutionally protected right to refuse treatment has been viewed by historical consensus as a bedrock legal and ethical principle of health care decision making in the United States (Morrissey & Jennings, 2006), it remains only one component of the universe of comprehensive public health and a socially just order. To support the flourishing of older persons and all members of society, aging and health policy must focus on all of the manifold concerns in people's social ecologies.

Policy theorists (Stone, 2011) have discussed trade-offs between values, such as the potential tensions between the value of liberty and the values of equity, equality, and security, in decisions about policy choices and the allocation of resources. Most of the time, those trade-offs do not surface as explicitly as theorists present them, such as the hotly debated topic of universal health care for all Americans, as opposed to the patchwork quilt of public and private benefits and programs that presently exists in the United States. Although the United States lacks any federal or state policy establishing a universal health care program, the concept of affording all members of the society equitable access to health care would, by virtue of its design, prioritize the value of equity. However, through the redistribution of wealth, it would also involve some infringement on individual liberty in the funding and allocation of resources to operate such a program.

Structural inequalities in society and inequities in access to care have spurred a counter-movement to the hegemony of consumerism and neoliberalism. This awareness has fostered critical theoretical perspectives that challenge the tenets of neoliberalism. Although these critical theoretical perspectives have moved slowly into the field of gerontology, their biggest impact in the formulation of a critical geronotology may be in linking the crisis of suffering in aging to public health. A critical theoretical public health perspective offers the most promising challenge to neoliberalism in bringing to the foreground the social and economic determinants of health over which the individual has little or no control. Although these determinants heavily influence the aging process and aging outcomes, individuals generally lack any means to change them apart from active engagement in political advocacy, which itself may be thwarted by the same determinants that impede the older individual in other arenas. The central thesis of this book—that our social and economic structures must undergo dramatic transformation to make our social, aging, and health systems capable of addressing the growing problem of elder suffering—is particularly relevant in discussions of policy solutions, as social and structural changes traditionally come about only as a result of changes to public policy through the mobilization of mass movements. Here we do not make the argument that all suffering can be eliminated or even controlled—a myth that Gregory and English (1994) have helped to debunk—but rather that we—both as human beings and as health care professionals and thought leaders—have an ethical obligation to relieve and reduce the risk of suffering through the development of effective policy and in the design of aging and health care systems, facilities, and services. We argue further that policy choices and decisions about system design should have the explicit goal of avoiding the heightening of elder suffering or imposing onerous burdens on elders that would ultimately result in greater suffering.

In this chapter and others that follow, we call for a critical re-theorizing of social structures and social systems with the goal of translating such theory into the field, applying them practically to aging and health policy processes, systems, and program design. Such practical applications would encompass not only removing barriers to elder flourishing, but also assuring conditions of living and dying that support health and economic security: freedom from intolerable and intractable pain and unnecessary prolongation of avoidable suffering, reasonable comfort in a welcoming home and community (using the term "home" liberally throughout this book), and palliative environments that affirm human dignity. Such conditions must be available, accessible, affordable, and acceptable across diverse neighborhoods and communities for all older persons in their pursuit of life goals, meaning, and fulfillment of agency.

B.   DEMOGRAPHIC TRENDS

The demographics of aging are critical to understanding the magnitude of the elder suffering problem. In this subsection of the chapter, we present relevant data, sometimes using different measures, as well as data analyses.

S. Jay Olshansky (Olshansky, 2015) has provided the clearest picture and analysis of aging trends in the United States, placing longevity trends in historical context. Olshansky reports that early achievements in increasing life expectancy, which measured death rather than health, were the result of middle to late nineteenth-century and early twentieth-century public health interventions targeting early-age mortality. During the later twentieth century, reductions in middle-aged death rates, such as from smoking prevalence and case fatality (e.g., cardiovascular diseases, diabetes, and cancer) reductions, also increased longevity, but to a lesser extent. According to the research analysis (Olshansky, 2015), there will likely not be another dramatic increase in life expectancy in the United States, as it would mean that most of the population would routinely have to live beyond age 110. Over the next decades, the age distribution of the United States and all other developed nations will shift from the typical pyramid to become increasingly rectilinear, becoming square by 2050. However, disparities in life expectancy and healthy life expectancy will likely continue to grow. Those who have the fewest years of education will experience the least optimal health trajectories (Olshansky, 2015; Olshansky et al., 2012). For example, Hummer and Hayward (2015) report that Hispanic older adults, who currently have a longevity advantage over white older adults, face a number of serious issues that could likely impact their long-term health and well being, starting with their status as the most socioeconomically disadvantaged of all older adult subgroups. Additionally, some may struggle with unresolved immigration status, inadequate insurance coverage, and ongoing disadvantages in educational attainment and income relative to non-Hispanic whites. The researchers (Hummer & Hayward, 2015) suggest that while these data have important implications for Hispanic older adults, who are projected to quintuple in number by 2050 (18% of the nation's population over 65, or 15.4 million), they also have significance for other disadvantaged older adult subgroups who may face the same obstacles to improvement in health and well being.

A Profile of Older Americans: 2016 (Administration on Aging [AoA], Administration for Community Living [ACL], & U.S. Department of Health & Human Services [HHS], 2016) (hereinafter "AoA Report") provides a snapshot of recent demographic trends in the United States and their implications. Based upon these data and trends, the sheer surge in the growth of the U.S. aging population clearly will challenge the capacities of systems of care, programs and benefits, and the workforce itself well into the twenty-first century.

i. Growth in older adult population According to the AoA Report, from 2005 to 2015, the older adult population, aged 65 and over, grew to 47.8 million people, a 30% increase since 2005. That number is projected to double by 2060 to 98.2 million (AoA et al., 2016; Mather, Jacobsen, & Pollard, 2015). The same 10-year period, from 2005 to 2015, saw a robust increase in the pre-65 age cohort: specifically, a 14.9% increase in the 45–64 age bracket of Americans, who will turn 65 within two decades of the data collection. The 85+ population, who made up 1.5% of the population in 2000, are the most rapidly growing segment of the older adult population. Their numbers are expected to double by 2040, from 6.3 million in 2015 to approximately 14.6 million in 2040. The frail elderly population is also expected to triple in the next 30 years (AoA, 2008). Women are living longer than men, as reflected in life expectancy and other data showing that older women outnumber older men 26.7 to 21.1 million, respectively.

ii. Racial and ethnic data   Trends among older Americans in racial and ethnic minority groups are noteworthy. Racial and ethnic minority populations increased from 6.7 million in 2005, making up 18% of the older adult population, to 10.6 million in 2015, or 22% of older adults. They are projected to increase to 21.1 million in 2030, or 28% of older adults. People of Hispanic origin, who can belong to any race, made up 8% of older adults in 2015. Among the 22% of individuals aged 65+ in 2015 who were members of racial or ethnic minority populations, excluding those of Hispanic descent, 9% were African American, 4% were Asian or Pacific Islander, 0.5% were Native American, 0.1% were Native Hawaiian/Pacific Islander, and 0.7% of people 65+ reported that they belonged to two or more races.

iii. Marital status and living arrangements   Older men are more likely than older women to be married. Only 45% of older women are married, compared to 70% of men. Less than a third (29%) of the total number of noninstitutionalized older persons live alone, including 9.3 million noninstitutionalized older women and 4.3 million men. However, nearly half (46%) of older women aged 75 and over live alone. In 2016, 34% of all older women were widows. Only 1.5 million older adults aged 65+, or 3.1%, lived in institutional settings, mainly in nursing homes (1.2 million).

iv. Income and poverty data   A Profile of Older Americans (AoA et al., 2016) also provides critical information about the income and poverty levels of older persons, as detailed below:

- In 2015, the median income was $31,372 for older men and $18,250 for older women. In the period of 2014 to 2015, after adjusting for inflation, median money income of all elder-headed households increased by 4.3%, which was statistically significant. Family households headed by people 65+ reported a median income in 2015 of $57,360.
- The major sources of income as reported by older persons in 2014 were Social Security and income from assets, reported by 84% and 62% of older adults, respectively. Those sources of income were followed by private pensions (reported by 37%), earnings (reported by 29%), and government employee pensions (reported by 16%).
- In 2014, Social Security benefits (33%) comprised the largest share of older adults' aggregate income, followed by earnings (32%), pensions (21%), asset income (10%), and other (4%). In the same year, Social Security constituted 90% or more of the income received by 33% of beneficiaries, 21% of married couples, and 43% of non-married beneficiaries.
- Over 4.2 million older adults aged 65 and over (8.8% of all older adults) were below the poverty threshold in 2015, defined as $11,367 for someone

living alone at home age 65 and over. This rate of poverty is statistically different from the percentage of older adults in poverty in 2014, which was 10.0%. In 2015, older women had a higher poverty rate than older men: 10.3% to 7%, respectively. Older persons living alone were much more likely to be poor than older persons living with families, 15.4% to 5.7%, respectively. The highest poverty rates were among older Hispanic women living alone (40.7%).

- In 2015, ten jurisdictions had poverty rates for older adults that exceeded 10%:
  - District of Columbia (15.2%)
  - Louisiana (12.8%)
  - Mississippi (12.5%)
  - Kentucky (11.2%)
  - New York (11.2%)
  - New Mexico (11.1%)
  - Arkansas (10.3%)
  - Florida (10.3%)
  - Rhode Island (10.3%)
  - Texas (10.3%)
- The U.S. Census Bureau released a new Supplemental Poverty Measure (SPM) report in 2011, which takes into account regional variations in living costs such as housing, non-cash benefits received, and non-discretionary expenditures, including medical out-of-pocket expenses. However, it does not replace the official poverty measure. In 2015, the SPM showed a poverty level for older populations of 13.7%. This rate was almost five percentage points higher than the official rate of 8.8%. Non-discretionary, medical out-of-pocket expenses, included in the SPM poverty calculations, accounted for a major part of the difference (AoA et al., 2016).

These data shed light on key economic determinants of health for older Americans, and they highlight vulnerable groups who are at higher risk of poverty, including older women, older adults living alone, and racial and ethnic minority women living alone. The higher SPM poverty rate is particularly important, as it takes into account medical out-of-pocket expenditures.

The Kaiser Family Foundation reports the following key findings in an analysis of noninstitutionalized older adult poverty in the United States, drawing on poverty data from the 2014 Current Population Survey (CPS) and pooled from the 2012–2014 CPS for state-level data:

- Close to half (45%) of adults ages 65 and older had incomes below twice the poverty thresholds under the SPM in 2013, compared to 33% of older adults under the official poverty measure, based upon a poverty rate of $11,200 in 2013 for an older adult living alone.
- The poverty rate was higher among women ages 65 and older than men in this age group in 2013 under both the official measure—12% for older

women versus 7% for older men—and the SPM—17% for older women versus 12% for older men. Among people ages 80 and older, 23% of women lived below the SPM poverty thresholds in 2013, compared to 14% of men.

- The official poverty rate in 2013 was nearly three times larger among Hispanic adults than among white adults ages 65 and older (20% versus 7%) and two and a half times larger among black adults ages 65 and older (18%). Rates of poverty for all three groups were higher under the SPM, with 28% of Hispanic adults, 22% of black adults, and 12% of white adults ages 65 and older living below the SPM poverty thresholds in 2013.
- In every state, the share of seniors living in poverty is larger under the SPM than under the official measure, and at least twice as large in nine states:
- California (21% SPM versus 10% official measure)
- Connecticut (14% SPM versus 7% official measure)
- Hawaii (17% SPM versus 8% official measure)
- Indiana (13% SPM versus 6% official measure)
- Massachusetts (16% SPM versus 8% official measure)
- Maryland (16% SPM versus 8% official measure)
- Nevada (18% SPM versus 9% official measure)
- New Hampshire (14% SPM versus 6% official measure)
- New Jersey (15% SPM versus 7% official measure)

In addition to the AoA Report and Kaiser data, findings from the *2017 Commonwealth Survey of Older Adults*, conducted in 11 countries, as reported by the authors in *Health Affairs* (Osborn, Doty, Moulds, Sarnak, & Shah, 2017), suggest that older Americans have poorer health and occupy a more precarious economic position as compared to neighbors around the globe. Twenty-five percent of older Americans experience economic worries and difficulties, such as lacking adequate resources for food and housing, as compared to the lowest rates of economic vulnerability in Norway and Sweden, respectively, at 3% and 4%. Among other key findings are the following:

- The United States had the highest rate of older adults having diagnoses of three or more chronic conditions, at 36%; in New Zealand, the country with the lowest rate, 13% of older adults had three or more chronic conditions.
- Older adults in the United States faced significant financial barriers to accessing care, with nearly one-quarter (23%) of older adults in the past year reporting that they have skipped a doctor's visit, a recommended test or treatment, or a prescription or dose of medication because of cost.
- The United States (along with Switzerland) is an outlier on out-of-pocket expenses, with nearly 22% of older Americans reporting they had spent $2000 or more for medical care in the past year, as compared to fewer than 10% of older adults in other countries.

• The United States has a significantly higher proportion of high-need elderly adults (43%), almost one-third (31%) of whom skip care on account of cost. (*High need* refers to having multiple chronic conditions or limitations that interfere with activities of daily living.)

C.   PERSONAL HEALTH STATUS, CHRONIC CONDITIONS, AND FUNCTIONAL
       LIMITATIONS

Older adults bear a heavier suffering burden than most other segments of the population because of the greater presence of chronic conditions and functional limitations among older populations. While these burdens affect personal health status and the capacity to participate meaningfully in society, they also have significant implications for the aging and health systems as a whole.

Although the prevalence of chronic conditions in older adults is well documented, including multimorbidity and functional limitations, recent studies have shed light on the compounding interactions of these trends (Osborn et al., 2017; Aldridge & Kelley, 2015). The most frequently occurring conditions among older adults 75 and older in 2015 were: arthritis (53%), heart disease (53%), cancer (32%), and diabetes (22%). In disability and activity limitations, 35% of older adults age 65 and over have some type of disability. Older adults with both chronic conditions and functional limitations contribute to the highest health care spending in the history of the United States, which spends more on health care than any other country (Osborn et al., 2017; Aldridge & Kelley, 2015). According to the Institute of Medicine (IOM) *Dying in America* report (2015), the combined presence of chronic conditions and functional limitations has had the biggest impact on high-cost spending:

> The impact of the combination of chronic conditions and functional limitations on health care costs is shown in Table 1.1. Of the $1.6 trillion spent on health care in 2011, 56 percent ($909 billion) was for the 14 percent of the population who suffered from both chronic conditions and functional limitations. The second highest category of health care spenders was those with chronic conditions only. This population incurred 31 percent ($506 billion) of total costs and made up 36 percent of the population. *It is clear from these analyses that although the presence of chronic conditions is a key driver of health care costs, the addition of functional limitations appears to differentiate a high-cost group within those with chronic conditions.*
>
> Consistent with the distribution of health care costs by chronic conditions and functional limitations shown in Table 1.1, the population with both chronic conditions and functional limitations is disproportionately represented in the top 5 percent of health care spenders. Figure 1.1 shows that those with both chronic conditions and functional limitations make up 72 percent of the top 5 percent of health care spenders while making up only 12 percent of the rest of the population.
>
> (Aldridge & Kelley, 2015, p. 492)

Table 1.1 Chronic conditions and functional limitations health care costs

	No. of people	%	Health care costs	%
Total population	312,514,999		$1,627,372,719,765	
No. chronic conditons or functional limitations	149,340,364	48	$186,301,532,393	11
Chronic conditions only	112,005,273	36	$505,675,587,925	31
Functional limitations only	6,222,515	2	$26,614,504,628	2
Chronic conditions and functional limitations	44,946,847	14	$908,781,094,819	56

Source: The percentage distribution of population and costs by chronic condition/functional limitation category was obtained from the Lewin Group (2010); total population and health care costs were obtained from the 2011 Medical Expenditure Panel Survey data (AHRQ and HHS, 2011), adjusted to include the nursing home population (CMS, 2014; National Center for Health Statistics, 2013; Sing et al., 2006).

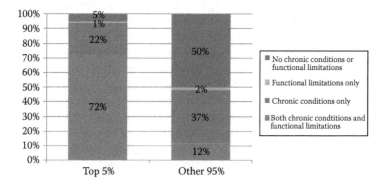

Figure 1.1 Total health care costs for the top 5% and Other 95% of Spenders by Current Conditions and Functional Limitations. *Sources*: The percentage distribution of costs by chronic condition/functional limitation category and top 5% / other 95% categories was obtained from the National Institute for Health Care Management (NIHCM) Foundation (2012) analysis of 2009 Medical Expenditure Panel Survey data these percentages were applied to health care costs from the 2011 Medical Expenditure Panel Survey data (AHRQ and HHS, 2011), adjusted to include the nursing home population (CMS, 2014; National Center for Health Statistics, 2013; Sing et al., 2006).

As cited earlier in this chapter, but worth repeating here, among 11 countries surveyed by the Commonwealth Fund in its *International Health Policy Survey of Older Adults*, the United States had the highest rate of chronic conditions among older adults 65 and older at 36%, as compared to New Zealand's lowest rate of 13% (Osborn, Doty, Moulds, Sarnak, & Shah, 2017). Along with Australia (39%), the United States also had a higher percentage of "high-need" older adults (43%), defined in the report as having multiple chronic conditions or limitations affecting activities of daily living, such as in the domains of shopping and cooking. However, importantly, the IOM researchers (Aldridge & Kelley, 2015) conclude that while older age may be a risk factor for higher health care costs, older adults make up the minority of high-cost spenders.

D. CAREGIVING RESOURCES AND RISKS OF ELDER ABUSE, MALTREATMENT, AND NEGLECT

Today's older Americans still rely to a large extent on informal caregiving systems (Osborn et al., 2017), leaving family caregivers to shoulder the burdens of care and perform complex medical tasks for their loved ones that often go beyond their capabilities and comfort levels (Osborn et al., 2017; Reinhard, Levine, & Samis, 2012). As these studies document, caregivers face increasingly stressful circumstances in meeting the demands of delivering complex medical care to their loved ones in the home. These demands, as well as financial burdens on caregivers and more broadly, a dehumanizing culture of care (Castro & Zautra, 2016), may also increase risks of elder maltreatment and abuse. (See Appendix A, Caregiving Resources.)

Elder abuse, maltreatment and neglect is a growing problem in the United States and one that contributes to elder suffering and burden. Estimates vary, but some researchers put the number at 1 to 2 million older adults who have experienced mistreatment (Bonnie et al., 2003; National Center on Elder Abuse). Types of elder abuse include physical, financial, psychological, and emotional abuse, neglect and exploitation. There is also evidence of polyvictimization among older adults, meaning that older adults may experience more than one type of abuse at the same time. Several federal agencies have responsibility for overseeing elder abuse prevention and prosecution including the Administration for Community Living (ACL), Administration on Aging (AoA); Adult Protective Services (APS); and the Centers for Medicare & Medicaid Services (CMS). The Elder Justice Act of 2010 (Pub. L. No. 111–148, 124 Stat. 119, Mar. 23, 2010, Subtitle H, §§ 6701–6703), and the recently enacted Elder Abuse Prevention and Prosecution Act or Robert Matava Elder Abuse Prosecution Act of 2017 (Pub. L. No. 115–70, October 15, 2017) are two important federal laws that aim to address this problem. Levels of funding for these initiatives will have a big impact on their implementation and effectiveness. (See Appendix E, Elder Abuse, Maltreatment, and Neglect Resources.)

E. SOCIAL AND ECONOMIC DETERMINANTS OF HEALTH AND INEQUITIES IN ACCESS TO CARE

The public health perspective takes into account the social and economic determinants of health and the multiple conditions and circumstances that shape older persons' experiences as they age. These determinants include food, clean water, sanitation, income, neighborhood, housing, education, transportation, health status, and access to health care services, among other factors. Educational level and socioeconomic status play a major role in determining health outcomes, including life expectancy (Olshansky et al., 2012). Researchers have reported:

> In 2008 white U.S. men and women with 16 years or more of schooling had life expectancies far greater than black Americans with fewer than 12 years of education—14.2 years more for white men than black men, and 10.3 years more for white women than black women. These gaps have widened over time and have led to at least two "Americas," if not multiple others, in terms of life expectancy.
>
> (Olshansky et al., 2012, p. 1803)

In a recent study of geographic health priority areas, or Medicare population "hot spots," with higher adjusted mortality rates for older adults that persisted over the 16-year study period, researchers reported certain characteristics associated with these "hot spots" including the following:

- Higher proportions of younger people
- Higher proportion of people from rural areas
- Higher proportion of non-Hispanic populations
- Higher proportion of residents with lower-income and education levels
- More income inequality
- Higher proportion of dual-eligible residents (i.e., eligible for both Medicare and Medicaid program benefits)
- More residents with poor or fair health even though they had higher health-related spending

The researchers concluded that health insurance failed to achieve health equity in these "hot spot" areas on account of social determinants of health, warranting a population health approach, and population level interventions.

Education also influences health and financial literacy levels, and the extent to which older persons may truly understand their treatment choices. Lack of education significantly hinders full participation in heath systems, and it may interfere with an older person's ability to exercise autonomy and self-determination, leading to a lower quality of life or reduced capacities to pursue meaning and purpose in later years.

Social and economic determinants of health drive inequities in older adults' access to care. Equity must be treated as a priority value in the design of aging and health systems. A public health strategy to improve both health and quality of life requires affirmative steps by sovereign nations, as well as states, cities, and communities, to assure equitable access to care through the non-discriminatory provision of health facilities, services, and goods (Gostin, 2014). Here we cite Beard and Bloom's description, from the 2015 *Lancet* series on aging, of what a comprehensive public health response to aging looks like:

> Thus, an effective public health response to population ageing must take into account the diversity in the health, social, and economic circumstances of older people, the disparities in the resources that are available to them, concurrent social trends, changing aspirations, and knowledge gaps. How can such a response be achieved? First, health needs to be viewed in a way that is relevant to all older people. In view of the likelihood of comorbidity and the centrality of geriatric syndromes in older age, a conceptual framework that focuses on functioning rather than disease would probably be most relevant. Public health policy for ageing could then be designed to maximize levels and trajectories of functioning in older age and the ability of older people to do the things that are important to them regardless of their functional capacity.
>
> This approach has several strengths. Fostering functional capacity can take place at all stages of older age, and before, and is a worthwhile goal even for the frailest or most cognitively impaired people. This process would also lead to a thorough consideration of the contextual factors—including issues of equity—that are so fundamental to wellbeing in older age, and will probably encourage the development of the more coordinated systems of health and social care that best address the needs of older people.
>
> (Beard & Bloom, 2015, p. 660)

The focus of this book—and our call for a comprehensive public health response to aging, aligns with Beard and Bloom's emphases on equity, contextual factors, and integration of health and social care. One example of such health and social care integration is the collection of data related to social and economic determinants of health through Electronic Health Records (EHR), an increasingly critical public health function. The design of EHR should allow for collection of both clinical and non-clinical information about the social and economic determinants of health. Such a systems design would involve extraction of social and economic determinants of health from EHRs and data aggregation. This recommendation is consistent with the 2014 Institute of Medicine report, *Capturing Social and Behavioral Domains on Electronic Health Records: Summary of Selected Domains*, which addresses how to capture social and behavioral domains in EHR, such as alcohol use, tobacco use, education, financial resources, social connections and social isolation, and race and ethnicity.

There is growing support for integration of medical and social data to improve population health. According to Laura Gottlieb and colleagues (2016), the goal of advancing population-level health through EHR social data extraction and aggregation will create opportunities for population management, as well as quality improvement and payment reform. This innovative approach to EHR may prove to be a promising direction in health care that will help to strengthen connections between clinical care and public health for older persons.

i. Health care spending and social and economic determinants of health   An overview of the macro health care environment within which older Americans must navigate, including trends in health care spending and escalating health care costs at the end of life, is critical to understanding the rights and needs of older adults in the United States and the design of adequate systems of care.

The most recent data on national health care spending as reported in *Health Affairs* (Hartman, Martin, Espinosa, Catlin, & National Health Expenditure Accounts Team, 2018) put total nominal U.S. health care spending in 2016 at $3.3 trillion, a 4.3% increase from 2015 levels of spending, and at 17.9% of the gross domestic product (GDP), also an increase from 2015 (17.7%). While there was a slowdown in spending in 2016 by payer for the three major payers (i.e., Medicare, Medicaid, and private health insurance) and by service (i.e., hospital care and physician and clinical services), aggregate national health care expenditures increased 3.5% or $354 on a per capita basis, reaching $10,348 in 2016 per capita health care spending, which represented the fastest rate of growth since 2007. Total out-of-pocket spending increased 3.9%, also the fastest rate of growth since 2007. This is an important trend for older adults for whom medical out-of-pocket spending may be a risk for impoverishment.

Highlights of the 2016 National Health Expenditure (NHE) data reported by CMS are summarized below:

- NHE grew 4.3% to $3.3 trillion, or $10,348 per person, accounting for 17.9% of gross domestic product (GDP).
- Medicare spending grew 3.6% in 2016 to $672.1 billion (20% of total NHE).
- Medicaid spending grew 3.9% to $565.5 billion (17% of total NHE).
- Private health insurance spending grew 5.1% to $1123.4 billion (34% of total NHE).
- Out-of-pocket spending grew 3.9% to $352.5 billion (11% of total NHE).
- Hospital expenditures grew 4.7% to $1082.5 billion, slower than the 5.7% rate of growth in the prior year 2015.
- Physician and clinical services expenditures grew 5.4% to $664.9 billion, a slower growth rate than the 5.9% in the prior year.
- Prescription drug spending increased 1.3% to $328.6 billion, slower than the 8.9% growth in 2015.
- The largest shares of total health spending were sponsored by the federal government (28.3%) and households (28.1%). The private business share of health spending accounted for 19.9% of total health care spending, state and local governments accounted for 16.9%, and other private revenues accounted for 6.7% (Historical NHE, 2016; Centers for Medicare & Medicaid Services, 2016).

The most recent Commonwealth Fund Report (Schneider, Sarnak, Squires, Shah, & Doty, 2017) puts U.S. health care spending at 16.6% of GDP based on 2014 data, a rate of spending that escalated over a period of more than three decades (1980–2014) and positioned the United States as an outlier among other high-income countries. If the 2016 NHE percentage of GDP data were used (17.9%), we would expect that the position of the United States as an outlier among nations would be that much worse.

The challenges in paying for health care and long-term care impose particularly large burdens on older women and their families. Hartman and colleagues (2010) have found pronounced gender differences in health care spending between women and men based on 2004 data. Total health care spending for women 65 and over in 2004 (58% of the elderly population) was $323.4 billion, or 61% of total health care spending for the elderly. Similarly, 70% of the 85 and over segment of the population were women, who as a gender accounted for 73% of personal health care spending in 2004. Per capita spending for elderly women was 12% greater than for elderly men; out-of-pocket spending was 50% higher for women than for men, 39% of which out-of-pocket spending for women went to nursing home care. Importantly, the researchers found that the biggest gender differential was in nursing home care, in which category women spent twice the amount men spent.

Over half of the beneficiaries of Medicare are women, and, in the 85 and older segment of the population, that percentage rises to 70% (Kaiser Family Foundation, 2009). With women living longer than men and experiencing higher rates of chronic conditions, the high cost-sharing requirements of the Medicare program and the gaps in long-term care coverage put them at high risk of suffering sizable out-of-pocket costs for their care at a time in their lives when they have fewer resources than men (Kaiser Family Foundation, 2009; Salganicoff, Cubanski, Ranji, & Neuman, 2009; DeNavas-Walt, Proctor, & Smith, 2009).

Turning to end-of-life care, estimates of spending in this area have been revised. Although per capita medical spending in the United States during the last 12 months of life is estimated at $80,000 (Osborn et al., 2017), and mean total health care spending in the last year of life is estimated at $82,911 (Aldridge & Kelley, 2015), the IOM *Dying in America* report (Aldridge & Kelley, 2015) analysis suggests that individuals at the end of life—of whom there are 2 million—account for only 11% of the highest-cost population (18.2 million). Put another way, almost 90% of the costliest 5% are not in their last year of life. People in the last year of life account for under 13% of total annual health care spending (IOM, 2015). Based upon these research findings, health care spending on end-of-life care is not the key driver of high health care costs in the United States.

In studies of variations in regional and hospital spending patterns on end-of-life care, however, researchers at Dartmouth (Goodman, Esty, Fisher, & Chang, 2011; Fisher et al., 2003a,b; Wennberg, Fisher, Goodman, & Skinner, 2008) as well as others (Yasaitis, Fisher, Skinner, & Chandra, 2009) have presented research findings that show the lack of a positive association or an inverse relationship between higher spending and outcomes or quality. In certain supply-sensitive regions of the country, chronically ill patients on average had many more physician visits in the last six months of life compared to the lowest supply-sensitive regions of the country (Goodman et al., 2011). Similarly, chronically ill people spent more days on average in the hospital and in intensive care in the last six months of life in certain regions compared to others (Goodman et al., 2011). In Manhattan, chronically ill patients were more likely to die in the hospital (45.8% of patients died in the hospital) as compared to other regions of the country, and spent on average 20.6 days in the hospital in the last six months of life, which was among the highest average compared to other geographic regions (Goodman et al., 2011). In a 2011 Dartmouth Atlas Project report on health care spending, Brownlee and colleagues (2011) presented evidence of continued, significant variation in regional spending on the Medicare program from community to community within individual states for patients with similar conditions. According to the IOM researchers (Aldridge & Kelley, 2015), these data suggest that higher levels of health care spending are not associated with higher quality care, as indicated by measures such as longevity, quality of life, or satisfaction.

The federal Medicare Hospice Benefit (MHB) program is the primary financing vehicle for end-of-life care for the aged in the United States (Hartman, Catlin, Lassman, Cylus, & Heffler, 2008). Financial burdens of end-of-life care that fall on public program financing and on families are only expected to continue to grow through 2050, especially with Baby Boomers aging into the oldest bracket (Banthin, Cunningham, & Bernard, 2008; Sisko et al., 2009).

The Medicare Hospice Benefit (MHB), enacted in 1982, has largely been a successful program (Mahoney, 1998; Lorenz et al., 2004; Waldrop, 2006; Taylor, Ostermann, Van Houtven, Tulsky, & Steinhauser, 2007). The MHB covers palliative and support services for beneficiaries with a life expectancy of six months or less who choose to enroll in the program. The National Hospice and Palliative Care Organization (NHPCO) reported that, in 2015, nearly 1.4 million people with a life-limiting illness received care from the nation's 4,199 hospice providers paid by CMS under the Medicare Hospice Benefit, with the average length of utilization lasting 69.5 days in 2015 (NHPCO, 2016). Nearly 30% of the patients served by hospice died or were discharged in seven days or less. Characteristics of Medicare beneficiaries who received hospice care in the same time period were: 58.7% Female; 47.4% over age 84; 86.8% Caucasian. The principal diagnosis was cancer (27.7%), followed by cardiac and circulatory ailments (19.3%) and dementia (16.5%). Patients with dementia on average received the largest number of days of care with a mean of 105 days.

A growing body of evidence indicates that hospice and palliative care services are cost-effective in various health care settings, including hospitals and nursing homes (Connor, 2007–2008; Morrison et al., 2008; Morrison et al.,

2011; Taylor et al., 2007). A study of hospital costs by Morrison and colleagues (Morrison et al., 2011) in four urban New York hospitals with more than 350 beds for the period between 2004 and 2007 showed that palliative care reduced costs among Medicaid patients with serious or life-threatening illness by $6900 on average compared to the costs of usual care. Study results showed that patients receiving palliative care spent less time in intensive care and were more likely to be referred to hospice. However, legal and cost barriers to accessing palliative and end-of-life care services persist. In order to become eligible for the MHB, regulations require that an individual be certified as having a life expectancy of six months or less if there is no significant change in the patient's clinical course.

Structural and systems issues may account in part for the suffering experienced by seriously, chronically ill elderly persons at life's end. Health care spending patterns, regional variations, resource use, and quality of care have important implications for the care of older persons.

F. INADEQUACY OF AGING, HEALTH, AND SOCIAL SYSTEMS,
    AND COMMUNITY-BASED SERVICES AND SUPPORTS

Unsurprisingly given the demographic data, U.S. systems of care across the spectrum are proving inadequate to meet the needs of older adults. In her book, *MediCaring Communities*, Joanne Lynn (2016) describes the serious failures of care systems in serving frail elderly persons, from community-based care to governance structures. The *Commonwealth Fund International Policy Survey Report* (Schneider, Sarnak, Squires, Shah, & Doty, 2017) provides perhaps the best lens for focusing on U.S. systems failures. In its most recent survey, which compares and contrasts health outcomes among high-income countries, the United States continues to rank last among these high-income countries in outcomes, including life expectancy. Despite spending more on health care than any other country in the world, our life expectancy ranks last, and administrative efficiency is ranked next to last (Schneider, Sarnak, Squires, Shah, & Doty, 2017). The 2017 *Commonwealth Fund International Health Policy Survey of Older Adults* (Osborn, Doty, Moulds, Sarnak, & Shah, 2017) in 11 countries (Australia, Canada, France, Germany, the Netherlands, New Zealand, Norway, Sweden, Switzerland, the United Kingdom, and the United States) reports that older Americans are sicker and experience greater financial barriers in accessing health care than older adults in other countries.

G. WORKFORCE GAPS

Serious gaps in the U.S. workforce will make it increasingly difficult to meet the needs of the burgeoning aging population over the next decades. Shortages of trained professionals in the fields of aging and health, such as gerontologists and geriatricians, are only part of this picture. The United States has also failed to develop a generalist-level workforce able to provide direct care, including community-based and humanitarian workers to deliver critical services to older adults and their caregivers. In this book, we bring generalist-level, including the generalist-level palliative care (Quill & Abernathy, 2013), workforce into focus as an essential building block of the overall workforce in aging and health.

H. CLIMATE ECOLOGY

Despite the scientific consensus on the threats of climate change, the United States has seen a retreat under the Trump administration from the more progressive policy positions of the Obama administration. Although the United States has taken steps such as withdrawing from the Paris Climate Accords since the tenure of President Trump began, climate change continues to have a real impact upon vulnerable older adults both in the United States and around the world, as witnessed dramatically in the latter part of 2017. Hurricanes in Texas, Florida, and Puerto Rico left many older adults in crisis situations that put their lives and health at risk, and in some cases resulted in deaths. The public health response in emergencies and disasters is critical to supporting resilience among older adults, especially concerning the provision of trauma-informed and palliative care services.

I. ASSESSMENT AND MEASUREMENT OF SUFFERING AMONG OLDER ADULTS

While there is no widely recognized or universal measure of suffering among older adults, there is robust consensus that older adults carry a heavy suffering burden as they age into their later years. Eliminating that suffering must be a goal of any approach to care and support for older adults. However, understanding suffering is enormously challenging, and some researchers suggest that the very nature of suffering makes it difficult to measure (Frank, 2001; Morrissey, 2011b, 2015). The *Lancet* Commission Report on palliative care and pain relief suggests a new conceptual framework for measuring suffering, called *"serious health-related suffering"* (Knaul et al., 2017, p. 1). As framed in that report, this measure may help capture suffering related to physically, socially, or emotionally detrimental illnesses or injuries that cannot be relieved without medical intervention. Diverse qualitative methods have also been employed in studying suffering. Studies of suffering among older adults using phenomenological methods yield rich descriptions of elders' lived experiences of suffering that may help to identify general structures of elder suffering experience (Morrissey, 2011a,b, 2015).

2.   Elder microsystem—frailty, multimorbidity, and dependency

Bronfenbrenner (1979) defines the microsystem as, "a pattern of activities, roles and interpersonal relations experienced by the developing person in a given setting with particular physical and material characteristics" (p. 22).

A number of components in that definition are relevant to the focus of this book, namely: setting, activity, role, and interpersonal relations.

The setting is a place of human interaction, and for older adults it can be the home, the nursing home, the doctor's office, the senior center, or a host of other locations where older adults may situate themselves in their everyday interactions. Bronfenbrenner's definitional elements emphasize the relational aspects of the microsystem in which persons interact not only with the inorganic environment, but with other persons in their everyday activities and roles. The environment is experienced by persons, not only in its physical and objective properties, but also as perceived by the person who makes meaning of her environment. This meaning-making activity and perception extend to the worlds of imagination and the unreal (Bronfenbrenner, 1979).

What does the microsystem for diverse elders of the twenty-first century, including frail and vulnerable elderly persons, look like? First, the magnitude of the problem that dependency creates for elderly persons is supported by the demographic trends. The gradual transition from a life of independence, drawing satisfaction from meaningful contributions, to one marked by a growing inability to care for one's self—and the social stigmas that accompany it—creates a crisis of identity that cannot be underestimated. Additionally, patterns of chronic illness, frailty, pain, and suffering pose increasingly difficult challenges for health care providers and health care professionals in serving older adults, in both institutional settings such as nursing homes and community-based settings. For example, nursing home residents who are frail and burdened with chronic illness live through a longer and somewhat unpredictable dying period characterized by increasing dependence (Lynn, 2016). Generally, frailty has been defined in the literature as an impairment of physiological systems, both quantitatively and qualitatively, and is characterized by factors such as weakness, weight loss, reduced activity and lower-extremity exercise capacity, and loss of energy, which have been shown to increase the risk of disability and death (Weiss et al., 2010). Chiu and Wray (2010) have presented evidence of higher rates of disability over time in adults with a diagnosis of diabetes, particularly for women, non-whites, and less educated adults. A study by Murphy et al. (2011) supported these findings in establishing a dependent relationship between functional disability and death. The researchers reported that decedents, as compared with survivors, experienced a rapid decline in functional ability in the months prior to death. Diedderichs and colleagues (2011) reported on a heterogeneity of indices for measuring multimorbidity and the chronic conditions that fit this definition. According to the researchers, multimorbidity is defined as two or more chronic diseases coexisting in the same individual. A common problem in older people, multimorbidity increases mortality risk, impairs physical and mental functioning, and negatively influences older adults' quality of life.

Many scholars have put a human face on dependency and chronic illness through rich descriptions and accounts of the experiences of older persons who struggle with waiting, loss of control, social isolation, and many other burdens of illness, as well as questioning their own identity (Lustbader, 1991; Charmaz, 1997; Morrissey, 2011b, 2015). Both Charmaz (1997) and Cassell (2004) have called attention to the dialectical processes of self and self-conflict that are inseparable from the experience of the illness itself. Cassell (2004) has also made a distinction of significance between disease and illness, defining illness as an affliction experienced and interpreted by the person that has meanings for the person independent of any disease category.

Patterns of suffering at the end of life are an important part of the elder microsystem. Part of that suffering may involve concerns about economic security, sometimes compounded by low literacy and self-efficacy when it comes to financial planning or decision making. While community members and professionals have some sense of awareness about the importance of avoiding unnecessary medical treatments that prolong elder suffering, the transformation of the aging and health systems is a labor- and time-intensive project in which change occurs slowly. Part of the systems transformation involves a paradigm shift from the current dominant biomedical models to a re-conceptualization of dying and conversations about dying, as well as a recognition of transitions to social roles of dying for frail and seriously ill older persons in stages of advanced chronic and life-limiting illness (Bern-Klug, 2004, 2006; Lynn, 2016). The 1997 book *Dying Well* by Ira Byock, a pioneer in end-of-life care, has been a major influence in helping to shift the conversation about dying to one that focuses on possibility at end of life—a perspective with which we are closely allied.

3.   *Mesosystem*

The mesosystem is the locus of connection between and among the individuals and organizations in the older person's microsystem. For example, an elder's health care practitioner may need to confer with her or his social worker, chaplain, caregivers, or family members in accordance with any applicable legal and regulatory requirements. Today, the aging and health care fields place great emphasis on improving care coordination for older adults, an effort that implicates the mesosystem predominantly. These initiatives seek to strengthen connections and communication among the providers and professionals in an older person's orbit, which at times provide fragmented care to older adults, given the absence of a unified health care system in the United States.

IV.   Elder-centered care framework

Against this description of the social problem of suffering and its environmental contexts, we turn to elder-centered care, one of the central organizing frameworks of this book. A major policy goal of the Affordable Care Act (2010) was to foster the development and integration of person-centered planning and self-direction in community-based, long-term services and supports (LTSS). Consistent with this goal, in 2014 the U.S. Department of Health and Human Services issued guidance for implementing Section 2402(a) of the ACA, spelling out standards on person-centered planning and self-direction. The extent to which a person-centered care approach has been fully and effectively implemented across the various home- and community-based services remains an open question. However, certain models of care, such as palliative care and hospice, have been person-centered from their inception and design.

The person-centered movement took root well before the enactment of the ACA. Carl Rogers (1961), founder of the humanistic psychology movement, in his earliest work identified several essential components of helping relationships, namely: unconditional positive regard, congruence or transparency, and empathic listening. These Rogerian principles, widely understood as non-directive in their essential nature, remain central to person-centered care today.

The person-centered focus gained traction in the 1960s and 1970s amid political and social movements to advance civil rights, patients' rights, women's rights, and independent living (Fins, 2006). The enactment of the American with Disabilities Act in 1990 and the U.S. Supreme Court's Olmstead decision in 1999 also stand as important milestones in this history.

In this book, we propose a shift from person-centered care to *elder-centered care* for several purposes: identifying and understanding the unique needs of older persons, developing an elder-centered health care science agenda (Wertz, Desai, Maynard, Morrissey, Rotter, & Skoufalos, 2017), and designing systems of care that will be most responsive to older people's needs. The differentiation of elder-centered care from more general person-centered care is an important step in the recognition of older adults and their human rights as older persons. The unique circumstances of older people warrant placing their care in its own context apart from the broader framework of person-centered care. The focus on elder-centered care emphasizes the unique role that older people occupy and makes it harder to lose sight of the respect they deserve as whole people with rich personal histories, a lifetime of experiences behind them, decades of autonomous determination of their life course, and an intimate, personal understanding of every phase of life.

V. Public health and global public health strategies for aging comfortably and palliatively

The focus in this book on elder health and well being incorporates a public health perspective. The World Health Organization (WHO) (1948) defines health not only as the absence of infirmity and illness, but as multidimensional—physical, psychosocial, and environmental, *"Health is a state of complete physical, mental and social well being and not merely the absence of disease or infirmity."* Public health looks at health through a population lens. Hence, measures of individual health, while still important to the overall picture of health, are not the primary focus. (See Appendix B for a description of categories of law and policy related to public health and essential public health functions and services.)

The 2015 WHO *Report on Aging*, which spells out the most comprehensive public health vision for older adult health and well being, calls for a comprehensive public health response to the aging of the population, providing the following context for the development of that response:

BOX 1.1 INTERNATIONAL LEGAL
AND POLICY FRAMEWORKS ON AGING

INTERNATIONAL HUMAN RIGHTS LAW

Human rights are the universal freedoms and entitlements of individuals and groups that are protected by law.

These include civil and political rights, such as the right to life, as well as social, economic and cultural rights, which include rights to health, social security and housing. All rights are interrelated, interdependent and inalienable. Human rights cannot be taken away due to a person's age or health status. Article 1 of the International Covenant on Economic, Social and Cultural Rights proscribes discrimination based on an individual's status, and this proscription encompasses age (15). By definition, human rights apply to all people, including older people, even when there is no specific reference in the text to older age groups or aging.

During the past two decades, major strides have been made in efforts to advance human rights, including those of older people. Several international human rights treaties and instruments refer to aging or older persons, enshrining the freedom from discrimination of older women, older migrants and older people with disabilities; discussing health, social security and an adequate standard of living; and upholding the right to be free from exploitation, violence and abuse.

THE MADRID INTERNATIONAL PLAN
OF ACTION ON AGING

In 2002, the United Nations General Assembly endorsed the Political declaration and Madrid international plan of action on aging (13). Three priorities for action were identified in their recommendations: "older persons and development; advancing health and well being into old age; and ensuring that older people benefit from enabling and supportive environments." Several key issues were flagged in the plan. These remain relevant in 2015 and are emphasized in this report. They include: promoting health and well being throughout life; ensuring universal and equal access to health care services; providing appropriate services for older persons with HIV or AIDS; training care providers and health professionals; meeting the mental health needs of older persons; providing appropriate services for older persons with disability (addressed in the health priority); providing care and support for caregivers; and preventing neglect and abuse of, and violence against, older people (addressed in the environments priority). The plan also emphasizes the importance of aging in place.

ACTIVE AGING

The idea of active aging emerged as an attempt to bring together strongly compartmentalized policy domains in a coherent way (16). In 2002, the World Health Organization (WHO) released Active aging: a policy framework (14). This framework defined active aging as "the process of optimizing opportunities for health, participation and security to enhance quality of life as people age." It emphasizes the need for action across multiple sectors and has the goal of ensuring that "older persons remain a resource to their families, communities and economies." The WHO policy framework identifies six key determinants of active aging: economic, behavioral, personal, social, health and social services, and the physical environment. It recommends four components necessary for a health policy response:

- prevent and reduce the burden of excess disabilities, chronic disease and premature mortality;
- reduce risk factors associated with major diseases and increase factors that protect health throughout the life course;
- develop a continuum of affordable, accessible, high-quality and age-friendly health and social services that address the needs and rights of people as they age;
- provide training and education to caregivers.

(WHO, 2015, p. 5)

The "active Aging" lens in this WHO report brings a much sharper focus to bear on the social dimensions of the aging process, and social and economic determinants of health. Importantly, the report touches upon the essential topic of supportive environments. This book emphasizes the notion of *palliative environments*, a term first introduced into the gerontological literature by Morrissey, Herr, and Levine (2015) in an article in a "Special Issues" edition of the *Gerontologist* published contemporaneously with the last White House

Conference on Aging. Building environments that are supportive *and* palliative, in the sense that the structures of such environments aim to relieve elder
suffering, must be a priority for the design of aging and health systems across
all settings.

Thomas Frieden's public health impact pyramid

Thomas Frieden's (2010) public health impact pyramid illustrates the impact
of context in supporting population health, noting the role of counseling,
education, and socioeconomic factors that have the greatest impact. "Public
health involves far more than health care" (Frieden, 2010, p. 4), as Frieden put
it so well. In his role as New York City health commissioner, Frieden advo-
cated for policy that would change structures to make individuals' default
decisions healthy—another level of population impact. For example, in New
York City, population-level initiatives by the New York City Department of
Health and Mental Hygiene (NYC DOHMH) to limit sugary beverage consumption and salt intake among New Yorkers, reduce fall-related hospitaliza-
tions, monitor health improvement through multiple other health indicators
and create age-friendly communities, serve as examples of policy interventions that aim to modify structures and set a floor for healthier individual
choices and decisions (Germain, Davis, Barbot, & Bassett, 2017).

Public health strategy for palliative care

A growing body of evidence supports the adoption of a public health strategy
for palliative care discussed throughout this book. The WHO public health
strategy for palliative care includes four key components: policy development,
access to essential medicines, education and training, and policy implementation (Stjernswärd, Foley, & Ferris, 2007). More recently, the Sixty-Seventh
World Health Assembly adopted a resolution calling for the strengthening of
comprehensive palliative care (2014), further affirmation of the widely recognized right to palliative care under international conventions, such as the
International Covenant on Economic, Social, and Cultural Rights (Gostin,
2014). Other recent research and policy advocacy have focused on building
palliative environments for older persons with serious illness and suffering,
including frail and vulnerable older persons (Morrissey, 2015; Morrissey
et al., 2015). The public health strategy for palliative care will play a pivotal
role in assuring equitable access to care for all older persons in the decades
to come.

VI.   Conclusion

The process of life-course aging in the United States today is fraught with
unnecessary suffering and risk. A political economy driven by dominant neoliberal ideologies has steered aging and health policy toward individual-level

interventions for improving health and well being rather than more holistic, macro-level solutions. The effectiveness of these interventions may be diminished by social and economic determinants of health, such as education, poverty, and neighborhood, which have an impact on older adults' health outcomes and over which older adults have little or no control. The adoption of a public health frame that prioritizes public health policy goals and interventions, population health management, and design of population-level and elder-centered systems of care holds promise for improved elder health, well-being, and comfort in the United States, even through the last days of life. To build environments that mitigate suffering and foster a range of flourishing experiences, it will be critical to change cultural attitudes about aging and to instill a recognition that virtually all older persons are capable of aging with dignity and comfort into their later years. A primary goal of this book is to begin that very process of social transformation.

References

Abbott, J.T., Glover, J.J., & Wynia, M.K. (2017, November 20). Accepting professional accountability: A call for uniform national data collection on medical aid-in-dying [Blog post]. Retrieved from: www.healthaffairs.org/do/10.1377/hblog20171109.33370/full/

Abramovitz, M. (2009). Women in a bind: The decline of marriage, market and the state. In A. Joseph & C.A. Broussard. (Eds.), *Family poverty in diverse contexts.* (pp. 26–47). Binghamton, NY: Haworth Press.

Administration on Aging. (2008). *A profile of older Americans: 2008.* Washington, DC: US Department of Health & Human Services.

Administration on Aging. (2016). *A profile of older Americans: 2016.* Washington, DC: US Department of Health & Human Services.

Aldridge, M.D. & Kelley, A.S. (2015). Appendix E. In *Dying in America: Improving quality and honoring individual preferences near the end of life.* Washington, DC: National Academies Press.

Americans with Disabilities Act of 1990. (1990). Public Law No. 101–336, 104 Stat. 328.

Banthin, J.S., Cunningham, P., & Bernard, D.M. (2008). Financial burden of healthcare, 2001–2004. *Health Affairs, 27*(1), 188–195.

Beard, J.R. & Bloom, D.E. (2015). Toward a comprehensive public health response to population ageing. *Lancet, 385*, 658–661.

Bern-Klug, M. (2004). Ambiguous dying. *Health & Social Work, 29*(1), 55–64.

Bern-Klug, M. (2006). Calling the question of "possible dying" among nursing home residents: Triggers, barriers and facilitators. *Journal of Social Work in End-of-Life & Palliative Care, 2*(3), 61–85.

Blevins, D., & Deason-Howell, L.M. (2002). End of life care in nursing homes: Interface of policy research and practice. *Behavioral Sciences & Law, 20*(3), 271–286.

Bonnie, R., Wallace, R., & National Research Council. (Eds.). (2003). *Elder mistreatment: Abuse, neglect an dexploitation in an aging America.* Washington, DC: National Academy Press.

Bronfenbrenner, U. (1979). *The ecology of human development.* Cambridge, MA: Harvard University Press.

Brownlee, S., Wennberg, J.E., Barry, M.J., Fisher, E.S., Goodman, D.C., & Bynum, J.P.W. (2011). *Improving patient decision making in health care: A 2011 Dartmouth atlas report highlighting Minnesota.* Lebanon, NH: Dartmouth Institute for Health Policy & Clinical Practice.

Byock, I. (1997). *Dying well: Peace and possibilities at the end of life.* New York: Riverhead Books.

Cassell, E.J. (2004). *Nature of suffering and the goals of medicine.* (2nd ed.). New York: Oxford University Press.

Castro, S.A., & Zautra, A.J. (2016). Humanization of social relations: Nourishing health and resilience through greater humanity. *Journal for Theoretical & Philosophical Psychology, 36*(2), 64–80.

Centers for Medicare & Medicaid Services (CMS). Historical national health expenditures, 2016. Retrieved from: www.cms.gov/research-statistics-data-and-systems /statistics-trends-and-reports/nationalhealthexpenddata/nhe-fact-sheet.html

Charmaz, K. (1983). Loss of self: A fundamental form of suffering in chronically ill. *Sociology of Health and Illness, 5*(2), 168–195.

Charmaz, K. (1997). *Good days, bad days: The self in chronic illness and time.* Rutgers, NJ: Rutgers University Press.

Charmaz, K. (1999). Stories of suffering: Subjective tales and research narratives. *Qualitative Health Research, 9*(3), 362–382.

Chowkwanyun, M. (2018). The War on Poverty's heath legacy: What it was and why it matters. *Health Affairs, 37*(1), 47–53.

Compton, B.R., Galaway, B., & Cournoyer, B.R. (2005). *Social work processes.* (7th ed.). Belmont, CA: Brooks/Cole-Cengage.

Connor, S.R. (2007–2008). Development of hospice and palliative care in the United States. *Omega (Westport), 56*(1), 89–99.

Cox, C. (2005). *Community care for an aging society: Issues, policies and services.* New York: Springer Publishing Company.

Cox, C. (2007). Social work and dementia. In C. Cox (Ed.), *Dementia and social work practice* (pp. 3–12). New York: Springer Publishing Company.

Cruzan v. Director, Missouri Department of Health. 497 U.S. 261 (1990).

Cubanski, J., Casillas, G., & Damico, A. (2015). *Poverty among seniors: An updated analysis of national and state level poverty rates under the official and supplemental poverty measures.* San Francisco, CA: Kaiser Family Foundation.

DeNavas-Walt, C., Proctor, B.D., & Smith, J.C. (2010). *U.S. Census Bureau, current population reports. Income, poverty and health insurance coverage in US: 2009* (pp. 60–238). Washington, DC: U.S. Government Printing Office. Retrieved from: www.census.gov/prod/2010pubs/p60-238.pdf

Diederichs, C., Berger, K., & Bartels, D.B. (2011). The measurement of multiple chronic disease: A systematic review on existing multimorbidity indices. *Annals of Family Medicine, 3*, 223–228.

Dijulio, B., Hamel, L., Wu, B., & Brodie, M. (2017). *Serious illness in late life: The public's views and experiences.* Menlo Park, CA: Kaiser Family Foundation.

Drummond, J.J. (2002). Aristotelianism and phenomenology. In J.J. Drummond & L. Embree (Eds.), *Phenomenological approaches to moral philosophy* (pp. 14–46). Dordrecht, The Netherlands: Kluwer.

Drummond, J.J. (2008). Moral phenomenology and moral intentionality. *Phenomenology and the Cognitive Sciences, 7*(1), 35–49.

Durkheim, É. (1897/1997). *Classical sociological theory*. I. McIntosh (Ed.) (pp. 212–232). New York: New York University Press.

Elder Abuse Prevention and Prosecution Act of 2017. Pub. L. No. 115–70, S. 178 (October 15, 2017). Retrieved from: www.gpo.gov/fdsys/pkg/PLAW-115publ70/pdf/PLAW-115publ70.pdf

Elder Justice Act of 2010, Pub. L. No. 111-148, 124 Stat. 119, Subtitle H, §§ 6701–6703 (March 23, 2010).

Estes, C.L. et al. (2001). *Social policy and aging: A critical perspective*. Thousand Oaks, CA: SAGE Publications.

Fins, J.J. (2006). *A palliative ethic of care: Clinical wisdom at life's end*. Sudbury, MA: Jones and Bartlett.

Fisher, E.S., Wennberg, D.E., Stukel, T.A., Gottlieb, D.J., Lucas, F.L., & Pinder, E.L. (2003a). The implications of regional variations in Medicare spending. Part 1: The content, quality, and accessibility of care. *Annals of Internal Medicine, 138*, 273–287.

Fisher, E.S., Wennberg, D.E., Stukel, T.A., Gottlieb, D.J., Lucas, F.L., & Pinder, E.L. (2003b). The implications of regional variations in Medicare spending. Part 2: Health outcomes and satisfaction with care. *Annals of Internal Medicine, 138*, 288–298.

Flatt, M.A., Settersten, R.A., Jr., Ponsaran, R., & Fishman, J.R. (2013). Are "anti-aging" and "successful aging" two sides of the same coin? Views of anti-aging practitioners. *Journals of Gerontology, Series B: Psychological Sciences and Social Sciences, 68*(6), 944–955. Advance Access publication September 10, 2013. doi:10.1093/geronb/gbt086

Fowers, B.J., Richardson, F.C., & Slife, B.D. (2017). *Frailty, suffering and vice: Flourishing in the face of human limitations*. Washington, DC: American Psychological Association.

Frank, A.W. (2001). Can we research suffering? *Qualitative Health Research, 11*(3), 353–362.

Frieden, T. (2010). A framework for public health action: The health impact pyramid. *American Journal of Public Health, 100*(4), 590–594.

Garbarino, J. (1999). *Lost boys: Why our sons turn violent and how we can save them*. New York: Free Press.

Germain, P., Davis, K., Barbot, O., & Bassett, M.T. (2017). *Take care New York 2020: Second annual update*. New York: New York City Department of Health and Mental Hygiene. Retrieved from: www1.nyc.gov/assets/doh/downloads/pdf/tcny/tcny-2020-annual-report2.pdf

Gonzalez Sanders, D.J., & Fortinsky, R.H. (2012). *Dementia care with Black and Latino families: A social work problem-solving approach*. New York: Springer Publishing.

Goodman, D.C., Esty, A.R., Fisher, E.S., & Chang, C.-H. (2011). *Trends and variation in end-of-life care for Medicare beneficiaries with severe chronic illness*. Lebanon, NH: Dartmouth Institute for Health Policy & Clinical Practice.

Gostin, L. (2014). *Global health law*. Cambridge, MA: Harvard University Press.

Gottlieb, L, Tobey, R., Cantor, J., Hessler, D., & Adler, N.E. (2016). Integrating social and medical data to improve population health: Opportunities and barriers. *Health Affairs, 35*(11). https://doi.org/10.1377/hlthaff.2016.0723

Gregory, D., & English, J. (1994). The myth of control: Suffering in palliative care. *Journal of Palliative Care, 10*(2), 18–22.

Guntrip, H. (1971). *Psychoanalytic theory, therapy and the self: A basic guide to the human personality in Freud, Erikson, Klein, Sullivan, Fairbairn, Hartmann, Jacobson and Winnicott*. New York: Basic Books, Inc.

Gutheil, I.A., & Congress, E. (2000). Resiliency in older people: A paradigm for practice. In E. Norman (Ed.), *Resiliency enhancement: Putting the strengths perspective into social work practice* (pp. 40–52). New York: Columbia University Press.

Hartman, M., Catlin, A., Lassman, D., Cylus, J., & Heffler, S. (2008). US health spending by age: Selected years through 2004. *Health Affairs, 27*(1): w1–12.

Hartman, M, Martin, A, Espinosa, N, Catlin, A, & National Health Expenditure. (2018). National health care spending in 2016: Spending and enrollment growth slow after initial coverage expansions. *Health Affairs, 37*(1), 1–11.

Havighurst, R.G. (1961). Successful aging. *Gerontologist, 1*, 8–13. doi:10.1093/geront /37.4.433.

Hummer, R.A., & Hayward, M.D. (2015). Hispanic older adult health and longevity in the United States: Current patterns and concerns for the future. *Dædalus, the Journal of the American Academy of Arts & Sciences, 144*(2), 20–30.

Institute of Medicine (IOM). (2011). *Relieving pain in America*. Washington, DC: National Academies Press.

Institute of Medicine (IOM). (2014). *Capturing social and behavioral domains on electronic health records: Summary of selected domains*. Washington, DC: National Academies Press.

Institute of Medicine (IOM). (2015). *Dying in America: Improving quality and honoring individual preferences near the end of life*. Washington, DC: National Academies Press.

Jennings, B. (1999). Liberal neutrality of living and dying: Bioethics, constitutional law and political theory in the American right-to-die-debate. *Journal of Contemporary Health Law and Policy, 16*(1), 97–126.

Jennings, B. (2016). *Ecological governance: Toward a new social contract with the Earth*. Morgantown: West Virginia University Press.

Jopp, D., Rott, C, & Oswald, F. (2008). Valuation of life in old and very old age: The role of sociodemographic, social, and health resources for positive adaptation. *Gerontologist, 48*(5), 646–658.

Kaiser Family Foundation. (2009). *Medicare's role for women*. Washington, DC: Henry J. Kaiser Foundation.

Knaul, F.M., Farmer, P.E., Krakauer, E.L., De Lima, L., Bhadelia, A., Jiang Kwete, … Rajagopal, M.R. (2017). Alleviating the access abyss in palliative care and pain relief—an imperative of universal health coverage: The Lancet Commission Report. *Lancet*. Advance online publication. doi: 10.1016/S0140-6736(17)32513-8

Krumholz, H.M., Normand, S.L.T., & Wang, Y. (2018). Geographical health priority areas for older Americans. *Health Affairs, 37*(1), 104–110.

Lawton, M.P., & Nahemow, L. (1973). Ecology and the aging process. In C. Eisdorfer & M.P. Lawton (Eds.), *The psychology of adult development and aging* (pp. 619–674). Washington, DC: American Psychological Association.

Lepore, M.J., Miller, S.C., & Gozalo, P. (2011). Hospice use among urban black and white US nursing home decedents in 2006. *Geriatrics & Gerontology International, 11*(2), 174–179.

Lorenz, K., Lynn, J., Morton, S.C., Dy, S., Mularski, R., Shugarman, L. et al. (2004). *End-of-life care and outcomes. Evidence report/technology assessment no. 110*. (Prepared by the Southern California Evidence-based Practice Center, under Contract No. 290-02-0003.) AHRQ Publication No. 05-E004-2. Rockville, MD: Agency for Healthcare Research and Quality.

Lustbader, W. (1991). *Counting on kindness: The dilemmas of dependency*. New York: Free Press.

Lyman, D.R., & Alvarez de Toledo, B. (2006). The ecology of intensive community-based interventions. In A. Lightburn & P. Sessions (Eds.), *Handbook of community-based clinical practice* (pp. 379–397). New York: Oxford University Press.

Lynn, J. (2016). *MediCaring communities: Getting what we want and need in frail old age at an affordable cost*. Altarum Institute and Joanne Lynn.

Mahoney, J.J. (1998). Medicare Hospice Benefit—15 years of success. *Journal of Palliative Medicine*, *1*(2), 139–146.

Mather, M., Jacobsen, L.A., & Pollard, K.M. (2015). Aging in the United States, *Population Bulletin*, *70*(2), 1–18.

Medical Aid in Dying Act. A.2383-A/S.3151-A, 241st N.Y. Leg. Sess. (2018).

Meyer, C. (1983). The search for coherence. In C. Meyer (Ed.), *Clinical social work in the ecosystems perspective* (pp. 5–34). New York: Columbia University Press.

Morgan, M., & Brosi, W.A. (2007). Prescription drug abuse among older adults: A family ecological case study. *Journal of Applied Gerontology*, *26*, 419–432.

Morrison, R.S., Dietrich, J., Ladwig, S., Quill, T., Sacco, J., Tangeman, J., & Meier, D.E. (2011). The care span: Palliative care consultation teams cut hospital costs for Medicaid beneficiaries. *Health Affairs*, *30*(3), 454–463.

Morrison, R.S., Maroney-Galin, C., Kralovec, P.D., & Meier, D.E. (2005). The growth of palliative care programs in United States hospitals. *Journal of Palliative Medicine*, *8*(6), 1127–1134.

Morrison, R.S., & Meier, D.E. (2004). Palliative care. *New England Journal of Medicine*, *350*(25), 2582–2591.

Morrison, R.S., Penrod, J.D., Cassell, J.B., Caust-Ellenbogen, M., Litke, A., Spragens, I., & Meier, D.E. (2008). Cost savings associated with United States hospital palliative care consultation programs. *Archives of Internal Medicine*, *168*(16): 1784–1790.

Morrissey, M.B. (2011a). Phenomenology of pain and suffering at the end of life: A humanistic perspective in gerontological health and social work. *Journal of Social Work in End-of-Life and Palliative Care*, *7*(1), 14–38.

Morrissey, M.B. (2011b). *Suffering and decision making among seriously ill elderly women*. (Doctoral dissertation, Fordham University). Retrieved from: http://fordham.bepress.com/dissertations/AAI3458134/

Morrissey, M. B. (2015). *Suffering narratives of older adults*. New York: Routledge.

Morrissey, M.B., Herr, K., & Levine, C. (2015). Public health imperative of the 21st Century: Innovations in palliative care systems, services, and supports to improve health and well-being of Older Americans. *Gerontologist*, 1–7. doi:10.1093/geront/gnu178

Morrissey, M.B., & Jennings, B. (2006, Winter). A social ecology of health model in end-of-life decision-making: Is the law therapeutic? *New York State Bar Association. Health Law Journal. Special Edition: Selected Topics in Long-Term Care Law*, *11*(1), 51–60.

Mullaly, B. (2007). *The new structural social work.* (3rd ed.). Ontario: Oxford University Press.

Murphy, T.E., Han, L., Allore, H.G., Peduzzi, P.N., Gill, T.M., & Lin, H. (2011). Treatment of death in the analysis of longitudinal studies of gerontological outcomes. *The Journals of Gerontology. Series A, Biological Sciences and Medical Sciences, 66A*(1),109–114.

National Center on Elder Abuse. Retrieved from: https://ncea.acl.gov.

National Hospice and Palliative Care Organization. (2016). Facts and figures. 2016 Edition. Retrieved from: www.nhpco.org/sites/default/files/public/Statistics_Research /2016_Facts_Figures.pdf

New York City Bar Association. (2017). Commentary on New York Medical Aid in Dying Proposal. Retrieved from: http://s3.amazonaws.com/documents.nycbar.org /files/2017130-AidinDyingNY_WhitePaper_FINAL_5.30.17.pdf

Olmstead v. L.C., 527 U.S. 581 (1999).

Olshansky, S.J. (2015). The demographic transformation of America. *Dædalus, Journal of the American Academy of Arts & Sciences, 144*(2), 13–19. doi:10.1162/DAED_a_00326

Olshansky, S.J., Antonucci, T., Berkman, L., Binstock, R.H., Boersch-Supan, A., Cacioppo, J.T., … Rowe, J. (2012). Differences in life expectancy due to race and educational differences are widening, and may not catch up. *Health Affairs, 31*(8), 1803–1813.

Osborn, R., Doty, M.M., Moulds, D., Sarnak, D.O., & Shah, A. (2017). Older Americans were sicker and faced more financial barriers to health care than counterparts in other countries. *Health Affairs, 36*(12), 2123–2132. https://doi .org/10.1377/hlthaff.2017.1048

Oswald, F., Jopp, D., Rott, C., & Wahl, H.-W. (2011). Is aging in place a resource for or risk to life satisfaction? *Gerontologist, 51*(2), 238–250.

Pincus, A., & Minahan, A. (1973). *Social work practice: Model and method,* Itasca, IL: F.E. Peacock.

Quill, T., & Abernethy, A.P. (2013). Generalist plus specialist palliative care—Creating a more sustainable model. *New England Journal of Medicine*, 368:1173–1175 doi: 10.1056/NEJMp1215620

Reinhard, S.C., Levine, C., & Samis, S. (2012). *Home alone: Family caregivers providing complex chronic care.* Washington, DC: AARP Public Policy Institute.

Rogers, C.R. (1961). *On becoming a person.* Boston: Houghton-Mifflin.

Rowe, J.W. (2015). Successful aging of societies. *Dædalus, Journal of the American Academy of Arts & Sciences 144*(2), 5–12. doi:10.1162/DAED _a_00325

Rowe, J.W., & Kahn, R.L. (1987). Human aging: Usual and successful. *Science, 237*(4811), 143–149.

Rowe, J.W., & Kahn, R.L. (1997). Successful aging. *Gerontologist, 37*(4), 433–440.

Rowe, J.W., & Kahn, R.L. (1998). *Successful aging.* New York: Pantheon Books.

Rubinstein, R.L,. & de Medeiros, K. (2015). Successful aging, gerontological theory and neoliberalism: A qualitative critique. *Gerontologist, 55*(1), 34–42.

Saleebey, D. (2006). A paradigm shift in developmental perspectives: The self in context. In A. Lightburn & P. Sessions (Eds.), *Handbook of community-based clinical practice* (pp. 46–62). New York: Oxford University Press.

Salganicoff, A., Cubanski, J., Ranji, U., & Neuman, T. (2009). Health coverage and expenses: Impact on women's economic well-being. *Journal of Women, Politics and Policy, 30*, 222–247.

Schneider, E.C., Sarnak, D.O., Squires, D., Shah, A., & Doty, M.M. (2017). *Mirror, mirror 2017: International comparison reflects and opportunities for better US health care*. New York: The Commonwealth Fund.

Sisko, A., Truffer, C., Smith, S., Keehan, S., Cylus, J., Poisal, J.A., ... Lozonitz, J. (2009). Health spending projections through 2018: Recession effects and uncertainty to the outlook. *Health Affairs, 28*(2), w346–w357.

Steptoe, A., Deaton, A., & Stone, A. (2015). Subjective well being, health and ageing. *Lancet, 385*, 640–48.

Stjernswärd, J, Foley, K.M., & Ferris, F.D. (2007). The public health strategy for palliative care. *Journal of Pain and Symptom Management, 33*(5), 486–493.

Stone, D. (2011). *Policy paradox: Art of political decision making*. New York: W.W. Norton & Company.

Sugarman, J. (2015). Neoliberalism and psychological ethics. *Journal of Theoretical and Philosophical Psychology, 35*, 103–116.

Sugarman, J. (2017). Psychologism as a style of reasoning and the study of persons. *New Ideas in Psychology, 44*, 21–27.

Taylor, D.H., Ostermann, J., Van Houtven, C.H., Tulsky, J.A., & Steinhauser, K. (2007). What length of hospice use maximizes reduction in medical expenditures near death in the U.S. Medicare program? *Social Science & Medicine, 65*, 1466–1478.

Vacco v. Quill, 521 U.S. 793 (June 1997).

Wakefield, J.C. (1996). Does social work need the eco-systems perspective? *Social Service Review, 70*, 1–32.

Washington v. Glucksberg, 521 U.S. 702 (June 1997).

Weiss, C.O., Hoenig, H.H., Varadhan, R., Simonsick, E., & Fried, L. (2010). Relationship of cardiac, pulmonary, and muscle reserves and frailty to exercise capacity in older women. *The Journals of Gerontology. Series A, Biological Sciences and Medical Sciences, 65*(3), 287–294.

Wennberg, J.E., Fisher, F., Goodman, D.C., & Skinner, J.S. (2008). *Tracking the care of patients with severe chronic illness: The Dartmouth atlas of health care 2008*. Lebanon, NH: Dartmouth Institute for Health Policy and Clinical Practice.

Wertz, F.J., Desai, M.U., Maynard, E., Morrissey, M.B., Rotter, B., & Skoufalos, N.C. (2017). Research methods for person-centered healthcare science: Fordham studies of transcendence and suffering. In M. Englander (Ed.), *Phenomenology and the social foundations of psychiatry* (pp. 95–120). London: Bloomsbury Publishing.

World Health Assembly Resolution WHA67.19. (2014). Strengthening of palliative care as a component of comprehensive care within the continuum of care. Retrieved from: http://apps.who.int/gb/ebwha/pdf_fi les/WHA67/A67_R19-en.pdf

World Health Organization. (1948). Preamble to the Constitution of WHO as adopted by the International Health Conference, New York, 19 June–22 July 1946; signed on 22 July 1946 by the representatives of 61 States. *Official Records of WHO, 2*, 100.

World Health Organization. (2002). *Active aging: A policy framework*. Geneva, Switzerland: World Health Organization.

World Health Organization. (2015). *World report on ageing and health*. Geneva, Switzerland: World Health Organization.

Yasaitis, L., Fisher, E.S., Skinner, J.S., & Chandra, A. (2009). Hospital quality and intensity of spending: Is there an association? *Health Affairs, 28*(4): w566–w572.

2 Philosophic science theory
Toward a phenomenology of a maternal cosmos in light of suffering

I. Introduction

The importance of theoretical and philosophical perspectives to the task of illuminating older adults' lived experience, especially experiences of chronic and serious illness and suffering, cannot be overlooked. Theory—especially philosophically informed theory—helps to make sense of lived experience and complex realities. The relationship between theory and practice is of critical significance, as theory may inform practice, and conversely, practice may guide the development of theory. In a sense, theorizing acts as a kind of practice of its own, such as in the systematic methods and practice of reflection utilized in phenomenology. In mapping the moral foundations of a socially just global ecology that gives primacy to suffering persons, we take the position that theory and practice remain inseparably entangled through ethical nexus. The ethical and moral demand for social justice contemplates the pursuit of theorizing, not for the sake of theory itself or its academic purpose only but rather in relation to our situatedness, sociality and solidarity with others. We make the radical claim that theorizing takes as its object the person, social group, or community to whom we stand in ethical relation, a social stamp, or community.

This chapter focuses on theoretical and philosophical frameworks in philosophic science theory, (Schutz, 1996; Embree, 2011), as well as theory of method. These theoretical perspectives may offer fresh insights into the life-worlds, encounters, and unmet needs of older persons as they move through life trajectories. We draw on the ideas of German philosophers Immanuel Kant (1724–1804), Edmund Husserl (1859–1938), Husserl's assistant Eugene Fink (1905–1975), Austrian-born social phenomenologist Alfred Schutz (1899–1959), French phenomenologists Gabriel Marcel (1889–1973), Emmanuel Levinas (1906–1995), and Maurice Merleau-Ponty (1908–1961), contemporary phenomenological philosophers Lester Embree (1938–2017), Michael Barber, and John J. Drummond, phenomenological psychologist Frederick J. Wertz, and ethicist Bruce Jennings. These theoretical and philosophical frameworks are not intended to be exhaustive grand theories that impose universal structures on experience. Rather, their presentation may challenge dominant paradigms and call for deeper reflection about salient issues of concern for older adults themselves, their caregivers, service providers, and communities, such as in the example of dementia care. In this chapter, we propose a social justice-centered theoretical framework within phenomenology, and we discuss its implications for aging, public health, and the interdisciplinary sciences.

II.   Phenomenology: Schutz's philosophic science theory— Theory of the cultural sciences

This chapter draws on phenomenology as both a science theory and a rigorous scientific method, and it positions phenomenology within Alfred Schutz's notion of philosophic science theory. According to phenomenologist Lester Embree (2011), Schutz's theory of the cultural sciences has four main structural components:

Schutz's perspective can be summarized as a structure of four levels:

- The bottom level is that of common-sense thinking and on that level there are the meanings that an action, relation, or situation has for an actor, the partner, and the observer in everyday life.
- On the second level is the model constructed on the basis of the common-sense constructs by cultural scientist in what can be called "substantive research."
- On the third level is the scientific science theory that includes the disciplinary definition, basic concepts, and methodological procedures of the particular science and these refer to the meanings or constructs of the lower two levels.
- And on the fourth level is philosophic science theory, which is theory of science in which more than one discipline is considered. Philosophic science theory is widest in scope but furthest from the concrete phenomena that are basis for the whole.

(Embree, 2011, pp. 8–9)

The interdisciplinary branch of philosophic science theory, or theory of the cultural sciences, that this chapter discusses has been influenced by phenomenological psychology (Wertz, 2005, 2010), phenomenological philosophy (Drummond, 2002, 2008; Barber, 2010a,b, 2011, 2012, 2013, 2014), phenomenological social work (Morrissey, 2011a,b,c), and phenomenological gerontology (Kolb, 2014). In keeping with the Schutzian perspective, Morrissey and Barber (2014) position phenomenology as a well-developed conceptual framework and qualitative method for studying, understanding, and describing human experience, agency, action, and decision making. According to Morrissey and Barber (2014), phenomenology seeks to provide deeper access than conventional natural science or quantitative research methods to first-person descriptions of experience, including shared experiences and their meanings. In contrast to the world studied by natural science that presupposes the physical thing as its object, in which the scientist is the only interpreter of experience, Morrissey and Barber (2014) elaborate further that phenomenology treats the social world as a regional ontology made up of first- and second-person perspectives, and it challenges the validity of the third-person perspective of the natural sciences and physical world. While phenomenology has been critiqued as anti-naturalistic and it is correct that Edmund Husserl, the founder of phenomenology, sought to rescue the science of psychology from naturalism by developing methods that were appropriate to the study of human experience (Wertz, 2016), it is more accurate to describe phenomenology as building knowledge through systematic reflection on the structures of experience (Morrissey & Barber, 2014; Wertz, 2016). This type of reflective knowledge gleaned through phenomenology complements the quantitative knowledge of the natural sciences, which historically have limited its fields of scientific inquiry into the material, physical world rather than subjective experience. Phenomenology brings a unique perspective to bear on the development of consciousness that encompasses the intentional relation between consciousness and the world, and the role of subjectivity in constituting and disclosing the world (Husserl, 1970; Drummond, 2008a,b; Wertz, 2016; Morrissey & Barber, 2014; Morrissey, 2018). The full recognition of subjectivity in the world may create fruitful opportunities in gerontology, public health, psychology, social work, medicine, ethics, and their allied disciplines for the fostering of hope and healing and for building a more sustainable and just social ecology for older persons.

A. *Role of moral intuition in cultural science theories*

An important starting point for discussion of cultural science theories relevant to aging and public health is the examination of moral experience and moral or ethical decision making, using the terms "ethics" and "morality" interchangeably throughout the chapter. Fields of interest include moral philosophy and phenomenology, moral psychology, and moral philosophy of law, as well as other disciplines. More specifically, our goals are to explore and examine the role of moral intuition, reflection, and deliberation in processes of moral reasoning, as they may help shape the understanding of older persons' suffering and the response to such suffering. We place the present inquiry in the larger context of a socially just global ecology in the service of older adults and in recognition of their moral experience and vision. For the purposes of this inquiry, we have chosen examples of that moral experience in serious illness, such as advanced dementia or at the end of life, for the very reason that such examples offer fertile ground for understanding what constitutes moral experience and moral decision processes for older adults. These examples present deeply contested questions and controversies in current moral and political philosophy debates about personhood and the obligations of a just society to older persons.

B.   *Moral experience and moral phenomenology*

The question of what is moral experience or morality, or what are moral judg-ments, is a foundational one in this inquiry. In Osbeck and Held's (2014) vol-ume on rational intuition, Giner-Sorolla (2014) defines a "moral concern" in a chapter titled, "Intuition in 21st Century Moral Psychology":

> For me, a useful working definition of a moral concern is one that takes precedence over other kinds of concerns in people's norms of what ought to be—that is, something we call morality should be spoken of as more important in principle than say, pleasure or self-preservation, even if in practice it is not always ranked so high; and (2) imposes the concern of a broader scale of social organization on a narrower one.
>
> (Giner-Sorolla, 2014, p. 340)

Here, the "oughtness"—or moral obligation—essential to moral concerns is made explicit. The author goes on to proffer the following definition of moral intuition as, "processes that provide information relevant to the moral decision quickly, effortlessly, and without awareness of the underlying ana-lytic process" (p. 341). This framing of moral intuition is arguably consis-tent with John Drummond's (2008a) account of moral decision making and action without occurrent or explicit deliberation. According to Drummond (2008a), the founding or presentational level of valuing is the descriptive objective sense and properties that belong to the experience and are tempo-rally prior to processes of emotion and valuing but occur as part of a unified experience.

We favor Drummond's (2002) account and treatment of moral intuition as evidence. The three dimensions of morality he identifies come from the perspective of moral phenomenology:

1 Everyday mundane, moral experience
2 Critical reflection on moral judgments and actions, both reasoned and intuitive evidence, and normative questions about *moral* agency (italics Drummond)
3 Critical and phenomenological reflection on moral agency with emphasis on agency (italics Drummond)

Drummond (2002) explains the transcendental perspective of Kant and its role in ethics. In the transcendental domain, a subject of experience encoun-ters moral phenomena and grasps, discloses, or constitutes the moral signifi-cance of things, situations, actions, and agents. Here, too, the transcendental perspective manifests at different levels, which has applications for the prac-titioner and older persons: consciousness as passive (i.e., sense of intentional correlation between value-consciousness and the value as apprehended which are viewed as independent of consciousness), and consciousness as constitut-ing (i.e., subject is active in constituting values and correlation between the

willing and the willed). For the purposes of this chapter, we frame consciousness in this latter sense of being constitutive in focusing on the older person
as moral agent, even in the midst of suffering.

C.   Levinas's sociality and ethical relation

End-of-life decision-making ethics has traditionally focused on the principles
of autonomy, beneficence, non-maleficence, and justice (Morrissey & Barber,
2014). However, the problems of suffering at the end of life, especially for
vulnerable, frail, and seriously ill older adults, oftentimes involve complexities that go beyond principled ethical analysis. The work of phenomenologist Emmanuel Levinas (1969, 1981), and his concepts of alterity, exteriority,
and infinity, illuminate the ethical and moral problem of suffering for older
persons and the nature of ethical obligation to the suffering older person as
other. More generally, through the work of Levinas, we begin to interrogate
how phenomenology as a scientific method can help us understand the problem of suffering for older adults. This suffering is grounded in older persons'
ordinary experience. For example, at the end of life, an older person often
faces the prospect of unwelcome and burdensome life-sustaining treatments
that unnecessarily prolong life or make the quality of life unbearable, or that
older person may simply encounter suffering as part of the experience of
being alive.

Levinas's notion of the "other" in ethical relation with human beings alters
conventional views of older persons and their identity of dependency—an
identity that has been constructed from a political economy perspective of
neoliberalism that gives primacy to the market and market transactions and
measures worth by capability of making profit (Estes, 2001; Cox, 2005). Estes
and others suggest that patterns of commodification, medicalization, com-
mercialization, and privatization contribute to the marginalization of older
adults within society and exacerbate their dependency needs. In a radically
different approach, however, Levinas establishes a notion of ethics as being in
service or "hostage" to the "other" by coupling it with concepts of welcome
and of hospitality. Rather than seeing the "other" as useless, Levinas encourages us to see the other as a person who needs to be valued, and even more so
because of vulnerability.

While Levinas's framing of responsibility to the "other" is an "undeclin-
able assignation" (Levinas, 1981, p. 139), meaning it cannot be assigned or del-
egated to another, he makes clear that submission to the status of the "other"
first involves a welcoming. In his two major works, *Totality and Infinity* (1969)
and *Otherwise Than Being* (1981), Levinas makes frequent references to meta-
phors of maternity and hospitality in describing the process of substitution,
by which the "other" as guest is welcomed and nourished through maternal
support (Levinas, 1969, 1981). Levinas sees ethical responsibility as thus motivated by metaphysical, existential desire. Metaphysical desire is distinguished
from lack or need, and it springs up only after needs have been satisfied by

"living from ... 'good soup', air, light, ideas, spectacles, work, ideas, sleep," or in engagement with the world (Levinas, 1969, p. 110). Levinas recognizes that a well-developed ego is a prerequisite condition for ethical relation. Only a capable and nourished ego can harbor a desire for infinity or the absolutely "other" and take care of an other, such as a vulnerable and compromised frail older person.

Ferreira (2006) defines sociality for Levinas as a surplus that excites the "same," "I" or self and draws the self to expose oneself to the "other." Responding to the call of the "other" is a movement away from the "complacent" (Levinas, 1969, p. 114) happiness of egoism and independence that evolves over the course of a person's growth, from satisfaction of needs and separateness from parents, to non-complacent happiness in sociality that involves no return or expectation of reciprocity (Ferreira, 2006). The "I" calls itself into question by welcoming the trauma of the encounter with the "other." This trauma of which Levinas speaks consists in surrendering one's self to the "other" in a radical passivity and vulnerability, prior to commitment, prior to freedom: a "pure susceptiveness" (Levinas, 1981, p. 138). Westphal (2008) takes the position that the trauma of self-transcendence that Levinas describes is inextricably linked with heteronymous intersubjectivity, in which the "other" occupies a status both elevated above and in conflict against the self:

> As trauma of identity, transcendence means that the Other is internally related to me. We find ourselves back at Hegel's notion of a relation "more like an identity than even the relation of faith or trust." I am who We are. Except that by virtue of the asymmetry of the relation we do not form a totality based on reciprocity. When in reflection I turn my intentional arrows back toward myself in order to recognize myself, to define myself and to choose myself in short, to say I, I discover the Other already there between me and myself ... This notion of being taken hostage, along with the notions of election and persecution, calls to our attention a second dimension of trauma. Along with my Identity, my Authority is decentered. I am called and questioned by the saying of the Other, assigned and accused, judged and found guilty. But none of these require my consent for their validity. Nor do I have any right of veto and deep down I recognize this. ... Finally ... the trauma of transcendence is heteronymous intersubjectivity because the Other, to whom and for whom I find myself responsible, is not just a law that comes to me from outside (formal heteronomy) but a command that contradicts my *conatus essendi* (material heteronomy).
>
> (Westphal, 2008, pp. 82–83)

The question of intersubjectivity and its constitution has been addressed in the phenomenological literature by Husserl (1913/1989) and Alfred Schutz (1957/2010). This question is critical to understanding elder identity as socially and relationally constituted. Barber takes up an analysis of this problem and highlights Husserl's and Schutz's differences on the question, particularly as they relate to Husserl's account of empathy. Barber (2010a, 2013) describes Husserl's account of empathy as involving a "transfer of the sense 'animate organism' from myself to another ... here meaning a practical recognizing of the other being as engaged with me as an interactive and conscious counterpart" (p. 4). Barber argues in support of Husserl's account for several reasons, among them the genetic nature of empathy. This character of empathy is fundamental to elder-other intersubjectivity, and it positions the carer—the person interacting with the older person—as also dependent on the elder. Through this phenomenological lens, we see that there is an interdependency in elder-other relations.

Richard Zaner (2002), in a very rich analysis of Schutz's intersubjectivity, reflects on the meaning of Schutz's "We-relation" and the significance of Schutz's writing on "being born and brought up by mothers" for understanding his conceptualization (p. 16). Zaner tentatively proposes that Schutz conceptualizes intersubjectivity and empathy as given in the primal Maternal relation. He states:

> We may then be able to suggest, albeit in the most tentative manner here, that being human is indeed truly a gift: being human is being gifted both with my life and the sense of myself (gift of life from pregnancy, birth); and later, 'gifts me with herself (through words; stories). Being born is accordingly constitutive of what and who I, any I, am; I am not merely, then, a "being-toward-death," but even more fundamentally a "being-from-birth ... I am indebted for my being to the Other (mother first of all), and responsible then for proper recognition of that and of becoming myself ... done within the nexus of growing old together.
>
> (Zaner, 2002, p. 17)

The implications of this analysis of Schutzian intersubjectivity for seriously ill older persons struggling with end-of-life choices and decisions are important. In the case example of a frail elderly person who is making decisions about her care and medical treatment, especially decisions involving refusal of treatment, the suffering person is the Levinasian "Other," making a moral claim upon human persons to serve. The "I" or the "same" is commanded to take responsibility for the elderly person, to take up her suffering. Using Levinas's maternity metaphor, the "same" receives the frail elderly person and is hospitable to her "otherness." Even though the elderly person is separate from the "same" in exteriority, they are intersubjectively related.

Some elements of the intersubjective relation that Levinas describes resemble fiduciary relationships, established in the law by one who places a sacred trust in another (Fentiman, 2003), such as the physician-patient, attorney-client, guardian-ward, executor-heir, and trustee-beneficiary relationship (Fentiman, 2003). The role of fiduciaries as advocates for aging persons or those living with serious illness is an evolving concept in the law (Fentiman, 2003). According to Fentiman (2003), central to the fiduciary notion is the obligation of the party acting in a position of trust to use his or her position "for the benefit of the other on whose behalf the fiduciary is acting, and not act out of self-interest" (p. 514). Pragmatically, we can translate the Levinasian moral claim of the "other" into a concept of fiduciary trust, in the context of aging. In serving the "elder other," the "same" (hereinafter self or fiduciary) is called upon not only to not violate the "elder other's" trust, but to actively substitute oneself in advocating for that "elder other." The concept of the fiduciary who gives priority to the concerns of the "elder other" aligns with Levinas's concept of disinterest. The disinterest that characterizes the self-other ethical relation in Levinas lacks intentionality, and instead roots the self's or fiduciary's movement toward the "elder other" in the desire for goodness (Gaston, 2003; Morrissey, 2011c). The submission to the "elder other" is not motivated by need or reciprocity. Within this ethical framework, the suffering of the frail elderly person opens up an obligation for selfless, charitable, and asymmetrical interaction, especially for the helping professional as fiduciary and advocate. Phenomenological literature also recognizes the cofiduciary responsibilities of members of the interdisciplinary team who serve older persons living with serious illness (McCullough et al., 2002).

In an article that focuses on ethics and the ethical subject, Barber (2010b) critiques Enrique Dussel's writings on global oppression in an area called liberation philosophy. Through this critique Barber highlights that the possibility of subjectivity made transparent in Levinas's ethics permits victims to become responsible for other victims. Barber (2010b) states:

> Though Levinas is correct that we cannot tell the other to sacrifice herself, which would be preaching human sacrifice, by depicting what is essentially, or to use the phenomenological term, eidetically, involved in confronting another ethically, he is at least intending to present a description, which he hopes that all—victims and oppressors, poor and rich—will be able to recognize as constitutive of ethical experience. ... Because of the eidetic nature of Levinas's account, victims, as well as oppressors, are summoned to responsibility, insofar as they are an "I," by their others, and hence it cannot suffice to assign them the role of the other only.
>
> (Barber, 2016b, p. 362)

Barber's analysis of blurred lines between victims and others can apply, for example, to seriously ill older adults residing in nursing homes, who may view the nursing home systems as oppressors and themselves as oppressed victims of structural problems that go beyond individual disease trajectories and illness burdens. For these vulnerable older persons, it is possible for them within their subjectivity to realize a responsibility to other vulnerable older persons, such as their fellow residents in the nursing home.

D. *Intersubjectivity and sociality: The pragmatist perspective*

An account of intersubjectivity and sociality, belonging to the school of prag-matist thought, has been developed by George Herbert Mead (1934). While Mead studied and cited some of the phenomenologists in his work, including Dilthey and Schutz, pragmatism and phenomenology have traditionally been viewed as sharing few commonalities either in philosophy or in methodology. While an exhaustive exploration of the differences between these two schools of thought is not necessary, it is important to establish that Mead attempted to establish a theory of intersubjectivity that has certain phenomenological dimensions. However, he broke with the phenomenologists in not accepting the self or the psyche as originally given in experience. Mead's work advances an understanding of self-formation that occurs through processes of social constitution. Mead's theory of symbolic interaction described above places a heavy emphasis on social roles and meanings that are rooted in action and practical problem solving. The centrality of social roles for chronically, seri-ously ill and frail elderly persons is key to understanding the meaning of their suffering experiences. Symbolic interaction theory has been used extensively in grounded theory research and in studies of chronic illness (Charmaz, 1997). For the purposes of this chapter, Mead's theory may certainly be viewed as a theory of the cultural sciences.

III. Social ecology of suffering: The maternal as possibility for older persons' agency, resilience, and generativity

We turn now to the role of older persons as subjects, actors, and meaning-makers. More generally, we examine the larger role of subjectivity and inter-subjectivity in shaping and constituting a global social ecology of suffering in the Anthropocene Period—an ecology in which older adults are embedded. The ecologies of suffering and aging are intersecting meaning systems that have varying salience at different times in the life course of older persons. We briefly describe the breadth of suffering in the Anthropocene Period and the phenomenological methods suited for inquiry into such experience.

A. *The character of the Anthropocene Period and its impacts*

A growing body of evidence supports the notion of the geological period called the Anthropocene, or human age, and documents the scale, temporal-ity, and detrimentality of the impacts of our human activity on all types of material systems—living and non-living (Jennings, 2016; Morrissey, 2018). The seriousness and magnitude of the changes to our climate and environ-ment are difficult to contemplate in our finite capacities as vulnerable human persons. Climate change patterns observed to date suggest highly disruptive and radical experiential changes, particularly in the destruction of habitats and homes, and the threats to planet Earth. From that destruction emerges the concomitant traumatic suffering and displacement of sentient creatures and human beings, including older persons. We have borne witness to such trauma and displacement on a small scale through the vivid examples of elder suffering wrought by the Atlantic hurricanes of 2017 (Dewan, 2017; Reisner, Fink, & Yee, 2017; Turkewitz & Medina, 2017). These examples demonstrate the breadth of concerns a phenomenological study of suffering must broach in the twenty-first century Anthropocene Age.

B. The person-centered focus on suffering: Fashioning a maternal cosmos and maternal systems of care

In adopting a person-centered focus—a person situated in an ecology of suffering, we seek to advance dialogue and invite deliberation about a public health response to the suffering of older persons that locates the very conditions of possibility for older persons' agency, resilience, and generativity within the primordial beginnings of such suffering. Older adults themselves have described the life-historical ground of their suffering as residing within, and indigenous to, maternal dimensions of existence, hereafter referred to as the "Maternal Ground." This *Maternal Ground* is disrupted through the experience of suffering (Morrissey, 2011b, 2015a,b). In a re-theorizing, re-symbolizing, and de-gendering of the Maternal, we locate the Levinasian ethical obligation to the elder other in a reconstituted Maternal Ground. That Maternal Ground—at the ethical nexus of theorizing and social practices—serves as both a wellspring for generativity and the foundation of a palliative holding environment for older persons who re-enact primordial Maternal experiences of welcome, unconditional loving care, and nurture. We call that palliative holding environment a *Maternal Cosmos*, built upon a spirit of nurturing Maternal care and liberatory practices that foster openness to diverse fields of experience and opportunities for agency and emancipation (Morrissey & Whitehouse, 2016). For purposes of designing care systems that respond to the needs of suffering older adults, we in turn call such systems *Maternal systems of care.*

Importantly, in a global context, the Maternal ethos, Maternal practices, and Maternal systems of care may act as a check on the kinds of human development of our ecological world that result in exploitation, deplete resources, or create intolerable conditions for the other, as suggested by Pope Francis (2015) in *Laudato Si*, for example. In this sense, the Maternal Cosmos and Maternal systems of care are imbued with justice in their social and relational constitution. As such, any cultural ethos or social code based on values of consumption conflicts with the paradigm of Maternal ethos and fidelity to the other.

C. Husserlian phenomenology and Fink's transcendental theory of method: Transcendence of consciousness

The unique perspective transcendental phenomenology brings to bear on the development of consciousness—with its emphasis on the intentional relation between consciousness and the world and human subjectivity in constituting and disclosing our world—makes it especially relevant to the project of gaining deeper access to experience of suffering and the transcendence of consciousness in its directedness to something other than itself (Husserl, 1970; Drummond, 2008a,b; Wertz, 2016). In this chapter, we focus on the development of consciousness in the older person—particularly consciousness *of* suffering. By applying the transcendental lens to older persons' existential situation, the present inquiry seeks to advance the knowledge of suffering in this twenty-first century—an era marked by environmental degradation, inequities across nations and populations, the threat of self-annihilation as a species, and, as persons and global communities, an inexorable march toward demise and death. Pope Francis eloquently described the need to care for "our common home" in his 2015 encyclical, *Laudato Si*, "The urgent challenge to protect our common home includes a concern to bring the whole human family together to seek a sustainable and integral development, for we know that things can change" (Pope Francis, 2015).

The arguments advanced here about suffering draw on Husserlian phenomenology (Husserl, 1970) and Husserl's notion of the transcendental. To unpack the complexity of Husserl's ideas, we draw on phenomenological philosopher John J. Drummond's explication of the ideas of the transcendental in Husserl's work:

> This looking backward and forward from the perspective of *The Idea of Phenomenology* yields the more developed sense of the transcendental, which is distinguished from the psychological in a three-fold manner: (1) transcendental reflection is not grounded in a region, but encompasses all regions; (2) transcendental reflection does not consider experiences in their being as real, mental events of an existent, psychological subject but considers them as possible intentional experiences of any possible experiencing agent; and (3) transcendental reflection does not consider objects simpliciter in their worldly, causal relations to other worldly entities, including psychological subjects, but considers them in their significance for us. The first respect is what leads Husserl to speak of transcendental subjectivity in metaphysical terms as an absolute being, but the point, I take it, of this language is not so much ontological as phenomenological. Transcendental subjectivity is characterized by a completeness that is lacking in psychological subjectivity, which is merely a region of the world, and it is not "relative" to the world but "prior" to it as the medium of access thereto.
>
> Transcendental phenomenology, then, reflects upon the transcendental subject in its achievement of making sense of the world and clarifies the essential structures of the various ways of making-sense of the world and, thereby, of rationality itself in all its dimensions. It is this distinction between the transcendental and the psychological and this understanding of transcendental philosophy that emerges for the first time in *The Idea of Phenomenology*.
>
> (Drummond, 2008b, pp. 202–203)

Drummond clarifies further that in working out these ideas about distinctions between immanence and transcendence, psychological and transcendental, Husserl resolved that "the appeal to the transcendental is the response to the problem of transcendence" (2008, p. 195). This resolution, so to speak, has important implications for the possibility for transcendence for older adults.

Eugen Fink, Edmund Husserl's research assistant, developed a theory of transcendental method in the *Sixth Cartesian Meditation* subtitled, *The Idea of a Transcendental Theory of Method* (1995). In applying a systematic elaboration of transcendental phenomenology to the problem of suffering for older adults in this book chapter, the goal is to explicate how transcendental methods constitute a moment in phenomenological psychological analysis of suffering. Transcendental phenomenology, premised on a pre- or non-existent transcendental subjectivity that Fink described as a constitutive source of the world, views subjectivity as unifying being together with pre-being. In particular, conceptualization of subjectivity requires insight into the process for achieving unity of pre-being and being. In this case, transcendental phenomenology can reveal the constitutive processes of suffering older persons as a subjective transcendental achievement. This chapter segment explores the processes of:

a   Constitution of suffering through disruptions or losses of the Maternal *eidos* or essential ground of subjectivity, and
b   Analogizing transcendental insights about world-constituting subjectivity to the generative character of the Maternal Ground that is the very condition of possibility for world constitution.

These constitutive processes involve a genetic approach to phenomenology, which examines life as a built-up, sedimented collection of experiences over time that fully manifest in the present (Fink, 1995). We note here that this approach has no relationship to biology or genetics. It is focused on the person and understanding the person's life history and experience.

C.1.   *Understanding of suffering in the natural attitude: Reflecting on consciousness of suffering*

The framing of suffering of older persons as a problem in phenomenological terms must begin with reflections on what is described in phenomenology as the natural attitude or mundane world we live in, out of which the portal to transcendental subjectivity opens. In the natural attitude, we find the intuitively given, pre-scientific life-world of everyday life, naïve and unreflective, although it does include existential positings. Even when we do reflect in everyday life, whether taking notice of psychological processes or thematizing meaning, the natural attitude remains straightforward. Whatever reflections and psychological intuitions take place in the natural attitude are neither sustained nor methodically employed in a critical, self-reflective, and methodical way. The natural attitude is a communicative, pre-reflective existence that concentrates its focus on the expressions of others in order to live in the life-world understanding of them as persons.

For the purposes of the natural attitude, the subjectivity of suffering remains unthematized and either unreflective or unsystematically reflective. In the natural attitude, suffering is treated as something that human beings passively undergo, oftentimes in isolation. Similarly, the dominant biomedical approach contends that suffering itself, especially in serious illness and serious mental illness, is an externally imposed affliction or even a disease that a person endures passively, without intentionality, and destructively to the self, identity, and agency. While aspects of this description may comport with aspects of the lived-through experience of suffering, it paints an incomplete picture. The passive view of suffering does not sufficiently account for the processes that constitute suffering through intentional consciousness or the relationship of suffering to the constituted social and cultural world. We often thematize our own or others' suffering, such as feelings of loss over the death of a loved one, a spouse, an intimate partner, a neighbor, or a resident in a nursing facility. However, consciousness of suffering escapes reflection. Here I call attention to consciousness—and, in this case, subjectivity—in suffering.

C.2.   *Phenomenological research*

The phenomenological procedures of the epoché—the impartial suspension of judgment—and reduction—within that state of impartiality, understanding the worldview of the person whose consciousness is being investigated (Giorgi, 2009; Wertz, 2005, 2010)—allow phenomenological investigations exploring and examining the suffering of older adults (Morrissey, 2011a,b,c, 2015a,b, 2016). These studies of suffering among seriously ill older adults, and their findings, build on incomplete knowledge about suffering in the current literature. The purpose of the phenomenological psychological reduction, which is a partial reduction, is to focus on and study subjectivity. Employing a limited epoché of the natural attitude, namely by abstaining from bringing one's own experiences to bear in validating someone else's lived experience, or existential positings, phenomenological methods help to access suffering in all its complexity including the role of subjectivity in suffering.

Studies (Morrissey, 2011b, 2015a,b; Morrissey & Whitehouse, 2016) suggest that suffering is a developmental process involving a disruption of continuity with the passively synthesized, common-sense world. This disruption or loss has been described (Morrissey, 2011b, 2015a,b; Morrissey & Whitehouse, 2016) as profoundly traumatic to the suffering person. That process is dislocating and alienating in its utter de-worlding, denuding, and de-habitualizing, and fundamentally antithetical to the habitualities of the welcoming home. In these suffering studies (Morrissey, 2011b, 2015a,b; Morrissey & Whitehouse, 2016), traumatic disruptions were accompanied by irreversible losses of a sense of home and individual agency. This trauma led older adults to move with intention toward a re-enacted Maternal holding, care, and nurturance, constructing a new sense of home in what Morrissey has called the "Maternal Ground" (Morrissey 2011b, 2015a,b; Morrissey & Whitehouse, 2016). The findings reveal the building up of suffering through a series of constitutive Maternal processes. Essential to suffering are these constituents:

1   Receptivity and welcome
2   Origin
3   Home
4   Holding and cradling
5   Relational intimacy, generosity, and nurturance
6   Empathy
7   Unconditional loving care
8   Well being
9   Generativity (Morrissey, 2011b, 2015a,b).

Losses of these Maternal dimensions of existence are a core constituent of suffering. Older adults' descriptions of suffering reveal that the Maternal Ground of life-world existence is a primordial source of meaning for them and opens up a condition of possibility for spiritual experience and development, recovery of agency, re-constitution of the life-world and its sense of meaning, and transcendence.*

Using imaginative variation—a practice in phenomenology of envisioning all possible conditions for a subject—it's possible to extend the analytic grasp of the Maternal Ground to all possible examples of suffering, and through such process advance the notion that the Maternal Ground is an eidetic— in other words, essential—feature of suffering for all human persons. For example, moving beyond the parameters of empirical research, the essence of suffering—its *eidos*—may also be captivated in art, such as in Picasso's *Guernica*. Art transcends the mundane world and the limitations of language in articulating the wordless presence of suffering.

In sum, phenomenological studies on suffering reveal its essence to be a moment of consciousness. Transcendental subjectivity, whether enacted on the part of a suffering person, a person recovering from suffering, or an artist who captures its essence in the art itself, allows a point of entry to understanding suffering.

C.3.   Explication of transcendental phenomenology, transcendental subjectivity, and transcendental theory of method: Relationship of suffering to the maternal

Phenomenological research findings on suffering among older adults can explicate the transcendental constitution of suffering and the relationship of suffering to the Maternal. Our aims here are twofold: to distinguish the

---

* See photographs taken by research participant Eduardo as an example of meaning and transcendence for one older man dying of COPD (Appendix G).

mundane from the transcendental while showing the relationship between transcendental and life-world suffering, and to clarify the whole analytic process of transcendental subjectivity grasped prior to its metaphorizing through its pure expression in the world. In this case, the subject of that inquiry is suffering.

Fink's (1995) explication of the process of transcendental subjectivity becoming self-aware and his mapping out of the transcendental theory of method to describe this process, as brought to bear in this chapter in the investigation of suffering experience, helps open up the black box of suffering with implications for the suffering of older persons. Fink (1995) frames the transcendental theory of method as the application of phenomenological methods to the activity of phenomenologizing itself. In such a project, Fink identifies three "I's" or layers in the process of transcendental life's disclosing itself and becoming self-conscious:

1 The naïve human being or mundane, "Human I" ("Human I") in the natural attitude, such as the naïve older person,
2 The transcendental "Constituting I" ("Constituting I") that directs itself to the world in its constituting activity and discloses the world to consciousness, and
3 The transcendental or "Phenomenological Onlooker," or "I of reflection" ("I of reflection") reflecting on the "Human I" and the "Constituting I," and who engages in phenomenological activity in the theoretical attitude, raising up out of constituting activity in the transcendental flow of experience.

C.4.   The "I of reflection" in theoretical attitude

The "I of reflection" does not participate in world constitution of suffering, only the constitution or production of scientific knowledge. The "I of reflection" is for our practical purposes the scientist. While the subject of phenomenological activity and the thematizing conducted by the "I of reflection" are the human person in various moments of everyday constituting life, the "I of reflection" is placed in the phenomenological reduction and takes up the theoretical attitude and theoretical activity. Fink (1995) is clear, however, that phenomenological activity in the transcendental reduction and its disclosure of constitutive becoming, is not itself constituting. In the transcendental reduction and reflection, the "I of reflection" experiences the loss of the world that "captivat[es]" (Fink, 1995, p. 42) and "restrict[s]" (Fink, 1995, p. 42) the "Human I," but never loses the unity of transcendental life (and being) and its transcendental ground. The "I of reflection's" loss of "*captivation by the world*" (Fink, 1995, p. 42) is nevertheless an essential un-worlding and un-humanizing. According to Fink (1995), it is only through this un-humanizing that phenomenological analysis of the constitution of transcendental life and being become possible, permitting a going-back to beginnings without antecedent, nor *a priori*. The "I of reflection" is in the realm of pre-being, coming before any form of existence or being. This is a paradox in that it is and is not a person. According to Fink, the various "I"s are the same and different in a kind of paradoxical, differentiated identity. In the movement from human being engaged in the world to the scientist who engages in reflection, to phenomenologizing activity, the "I of reflection" loses his or her positionality in the world.

C.5.   *Primary and secondary enworlding: Transcendence*

Although the theoretical splitting of the "I" into the non-participant "I of reflection" and the "Constituting I" results in antithetically opposite transcendental movements directionally, Fink explains that these dialectical movements ultimately result in different types of "enworlding" (Fink, 1995, p. 106):

1   The primary "enworlding" or embedding of the constituting subject as the human person—in this case, older person—in the mundane world (along with constituted mundane objects); and
2   The secondary "enworlding" of the non-participant "I of reflection" who is swept back into the world and humanized.

   The implications of this secondary enworlding are twofold: the "I of reflection" (1) returns to the passively synthesized, mundane world in a movement that unifies transcendental life, transforming a self-conscious awareness of the self-constitution of transcendental subjectivity into the human person as mundane world subject; and (2) now engages in the activity of transcending in the mundane world itself, expressing in mundane language the insights gained about the processes of constituting subjectivity and setting the stage to practice phenomenology as a science in the world, engaging with other scholars as a human being among others. The iterative patterns of movement and convergence of the three I's in the passively synthesized, mundane world chart a circle of beginnings and endings that flow seamlessly into each other (Fink, 1995).

   Several moments in the world-constituting process described by Fink reveal layered dimensions of discontinuity, disruption, and traumatic encounter, and, at the same time, bring about unity and self-clarification. These dialectical movements and moments may be analogized to the experience of the primordial Maternal relation, and its temporalizing in birth and human development, as described in the psychological literature (Wertz, 1981), through processes of discontinuity and disruption, and may be placed in the larger context of the analogizing of transcendental subjectivity to the *eidos* or essence of the Maternal Ground and its processes of generativity.

C.6.   Eidetic analysis: Mundane and transcendental levels

Fink (1995) identifies two levels of eidetic analysis in his explication of tran-scendental subjectivity: the *eidos* in the mundane, pre-given world and the transcendental *eidos*. This type of mundane eidetic knowledge is a thematiza-tion and appropriation of an *a priori*, unthematized knowing already in the possession of the mundane subject that is objectivated through phenomeno-logical activity.

At the mundane level of existence, where we are not in the transcendental reduction but in the phenomenological psychological reduction that reduces only objects, the constitution of the meaning structures of suffering is dis-closed. Here, reflection by the "I of reflection" and a shift in attitude reveal dimensions of suffering that are not given in the natural attitude. Meanings of suffering as they appear in the world may be pre-reflective and unthema-tized through sedimentation of past experiences built up in the world. It is exactly through this type of passive synthesis that meanings of the Maternal Ground have emerged in descriptions of suffering experience by study partici-pants in phenomenological studies of suffering (Morrissey, 2011b, 2015a,b; Morrissey & Whitehouse, 2016), disclosing the Maternal Ground as an essen-tial constituent of suffering.

C.7.   Suffering and the intentional spectrum: Transcendental eidos

In contrast to the mundane *eidos*, the transcendental *eidos* has no such ante-cedency in an unthematized knowing of the pre-given world, but rather is first objectivated by an act of ideation in phenomenologizing. The eidetic ide-ation process of the "I of reflection" reveals itself in the mode of pre-being. Fink describes this process as, "ontifying ... *onti-[fying] the 'pre-existent' life-processes of transcendental subjectivity*" (Fink, 1995, p. 76).

We argue that suffering is necessarily constituted and disclosed through intentional processes, as suffering is a form of being known intuitively in the pre-given world in implicit horizons that go beyond the psychological sub-ject. Turning to phenomenology and its cognitive practices as a science, the transcendental reduction discloses suffering as a unity that is productively constituted, having come to be in the mundane world through processes of constituting subjectivity in what Fink calls "end-constituted objectiveness" (Fink, 1995, p. 74). In other words, according to the transcendental theory of subjectivity, what appears in the mundane world is already constituted, the end products as Fink describes them of transcendental subjectivity's constitut-ing activity. In the transcendental reduction, the world and everything in it is bracketed and the "I of reflection" is able to reflect systematically in the theo-retical attitude on how suffering is constituted through those processes going back to its primordial first origin that has no antecedent in any form of being.

Systematic reflections of phenomenological methods in studies of suf-fering (Morrissey, 2011b, 2015a,b) disclose that suffering has its beginnings in the constitutive processes of the Maternal Ground, without which suffering would not be possible. In these studies, the Maternal has been interrogated as it has appeared in the context of suffering—*the Maternal* as the "thing itself" (Husserl, 1970; Wertz, 2010) or concrete reality appearing in the temporal horizons of suffering experience as an independent ground of possibility for the world. The contours of the Maternal Ground are mapped out in dialectical movements and horizonal entanglements with suffering experience, from its first constitutive processes through its full disclosure in the mundane world as pre-given. In this mapping-out of the architecture of the Maternal Ground, a clear distinction is made between the Maternal as a general and universal human experience, and what we more commonly describe as "mothering," meaning the parenting of a child by a biological mother or mother surrogate, although this is not excluded from the general. Study findings draw upon a broader concept of the Maternal that describes a certain pre-given condition of possibility in lived-through ordinary experiences of all people, of all genders, even if they have never been biological mothers, surrogates, or parents. Framed and envisioned as transcendental *eidos*, the Maternal is a symbol of generativity and pure possibility that is invariant and makes itself manifest in the world in a manifold of appearances.

The concept of the Maternal Ground builds and expands on earlier work in psychoanalysis and developmental psychology (Morrissey, 2011c; Wertz et al., 2011). Morrissey frames the Maternal as a pre-given condition of possibility in the lived world not confined to the sphere of influence of the mother figure alone, or to a dyadic, one-on-one relationship, but as belonging to a larger social ecology that extends to animals and non-human things, such as the ground we walk on that supports us, the food we eat that nurtures us, or music that holds us, soothes us, and gives us comfort. This expansion of consciousness of the Maternal as a ground of the intentional structure of suffering manifests itself in re-enactments of the Maternal through Maternal care-seeking behavior. More generally, the structure of the Maternal as articulated forms a ground for a suffering person's subject-world intentional connection, as situated against changing horizons and contexts. The Maternal provides a medium through which one can recover the full life of consciousness and engagement with the world. As a ground of suffering experience, the Maternal also creates the conditions for human dignity and irreducible personhood, from time in the womb to the worlding we experience at birth. It provides the setting for the processes of our becoming from birth to death, and in our undertaking of reflective moral action and creative freedom, as expressed so eloquently by Gabriel Marcel (1949, 1964).

IV.   Implications of theorizing for older adults' agency, resilience, and generativity: The example of dementia

Theorizing about subjectivity in relation to suffering helps illuminate the meaning of suffering for older persons, especially as such meanings concern the Maternal dimensions of existence. Drawing on these phenomenological treatments of Schutz's philosophic cultural science theory and Fink's transcendental theory of method, an ethical Maternal paradigm emerges as a ground to give social and cultural context for older persons' positioning, signifying, and possibilizing. The Maternal paradigm resists oppressive structures and reconstitutes power and social practices for the older person. Through engagement and collaborative practices that build community and solidarity, the Maternal presents itself as a cosmos, an affordance and a threshold of openness to experiences that can foster older persons' agency, generativity, hope, and dialectical processes of disruption and dialogue.

We now place this theorizing in the context of the example of dementia and its framing as a public health problem.

A. Framing the problem of dementia: Public health perspective

The personal and public health challenges of the experience of dementia— a conspicuous example of loss of the Maternal Grand in the suffering of older persons—will escalate as global demographics shift to include a great number of older people (World Health Organization, 2012; Alzheimer's Disease International, 2013; Livingston et al., 2017). Although dementia is a major contributor to disability and dependency among older people, the widespread lack of understanding about the condition results in stigmatization. As a result, people with dementia encounter barriers to timely, effective supportive services that could promote their health and well being, as well as their functional independence, quality of life, and flourishing. Such services could also reduce the caregiving demands placed on family and health care providers and to that extent would represent a fiscally prudent investment for society. A public health perspective on dementia emphasizes the systems and social contexts of high-quality, sustainable care and clarifies the social and economic determinants of dementia and the community capabilities related to improving quality of life (Chin, Negash, & Hamilton, 2011). Currently, a better understanding of comorbid conditions and risk factors that often accompany dementia is leading to social and behavioral, as well as medical, interventions to reduce prevalence and delay onset of disabling symptoms. Accumulating evidence suggests that public health interventions will be essential in meeting the needs of people, families, and the social challenges that dementia poses (Callahan, et al., 2014).

B. Evidence-based public health strategies to build capacities and environments

Medical supports and interventions must be accompanied by enhanced capacity-building across the health care infrastructure and improved systems of long-term dementia care, home care supportive services, community-based programs, and innovative dementia care facilities. This home, community, and institutional capacity-building should have a palliative orientation, targeting the design of palliative, Maternal environments and improved systems of dementia care. However, building an enhanced caregiving infrastructure for the future will be challenging. The already-high financial costs of dementia will continue until demographic trends might bend the dementia cost curve downward. Moreover, the lack of adequate long-term care social insurance in the United States threatens to produce an unjust disparity between the dementia care available to affluent, private-pay patients, and families left to manage costs of care on their own. Making necessary improvements in the caregiving infrastructure will require comprehensive public health prepared-ness and planning efforts. These efforts include: (1) monitoring the problem through ongoing epidemiological research; (2) supporting clinical research to improve therapeutic options; (3) supporting psychological, nursing and social work research to improve the modalities of dementia caregiving, along with creating settings of care that enhance quality of life and encourage continued social function; (4) planning and pursuing policy efforts involving relevant stakeholders, civil society groups, and the general public; (5) setting priori-ties for action; (6) improving inter-sectoral collaboration; (7) committing to public policies and to financing that provide formal and informal caregiving support in the community.

Research to understand, prevent, and treat the neurological causes of dementia is often more salient in public discussions than the social, insti-tutional, and contextual dimensions in which the impairments of dementia arise and in which ethical and humane caregiving responses must be made. A primarily medical, pharmacological response strategy, as important as those fields are, should not overshadow a social and public health orientation. Dementia is a public health problem not solely because it affects a popula-tion or a large number of people. It is a public health problem because it calls for a public health response: the development of environments of care and building community and institutional capacity to provide care systems and models that promote dignity, quality of life, and the preservation of personal agency and relational interaction during the course of the dementing illness (Whitehouse & George, 2015).

A public health focus can bring a needed balance among these perspectives into the social and health policy discussion, which will become even more important in the coming years. The incidence of dementia increases with age, bringing with it increasingly heavy care needs for the affected person over the course of many years (Schulz & Martire, 2004). Yet in some popu-lations the incidence of dementia is declining, a development that may be reasonably interpreted as a result of public health interventions (Whitehouse & George, 2015). Moreover, reductive approaches that define dementia in terms of neurological models have been challenged by more complex, multi-factorial understandings of the dementia syndrome (National Institutes of Health, 2013).

For the purposes of this chapter, we limit our focus to the phenomenon of prolonged, progressive cognitive impairment closely associated with aging, such as Alzheimer's disease (AD), considered the most prevalent type of dementia.

In sum, scientifically and conceptually, dementia is a dynamic arena today. The causes of AD are uncertain, but researchers believe multiple genetic and environmental factors play a role (National Institutes of Health, 2013). The relationship between diagnostic neuropathology and cognitive and behavioral symptoms is variable and not well understood. Furthermore, there is a distinct movement toward early, pre-symptomatic intervention and prevention, as progress with post-symptomatic medical treatment has been disappointing (Le Couteur, Doust, Creasey, & Brayne, 2013). Here, the difference between a clinical-person approach and a social public health approach is significant. In the context of limited resources and competition for support and public attention, expensive strategies like vaccination, given to people without any symptoms, can well eclipse alternative public health strategies aimed at the social and behavioral risk factors linked to dementia, such as developing education campaigns to increase exercise and healthy eating (D'Altona, Hunter, Whitehouse, Brayne, & George, 2014; Whitehouse & George, 2015).

Thus, there is considerable ferment and substantive disagreement over not only clinical management and financing issues, but also inevitably over broader ethical values (Le Couteur et al., 2013). Medical and public health approaches come from different directions and have varying policy implications. Is Alzheimer's a distinctive disease, or multiple diseases, of the brain, or is it a spectrum disorder with multiple epigenetic, environmental, and social determinants? Is a neuro-pharmacological strategy best suited to primary and secondary prevention, or is a social and public health prevention strategy a more effective approach? There is a pressing need to address how to manage the translational elements of ongoing medical and neurological research on AD. Also, translational work is needed to bring the best social, communicative, and psychological research to bear on the setting and practice of long-term dementia care (UK Health Forum, 2014).

C. *Ethical issues*

The exigencies of supporting persons with dementia and those who provide care and assistance to them pose numerous ethical questions to policy makers and health professionals. The symptomatic profile typical of dementia represents a kind of perfect ethical storm. The ethical dilemmas of dementia care put pressure on our sense of obligation to care for family, the duties of health care professionals, and the capacity of long-term care facilities to provide high-quality services to meet the special needs of dementia patients (Mor et al., 2004). A public health perspective locates ethical questions within the structure and functioning of institutions themselves—research institutions, acute and long-term health care institutions, and social support structures within communities at the national, state, and local levels. This perspective sheds a new light on key ethical issues including human rights, respect for dignity, maintenance of autonomy, quality of life, relief of suffering, and stewardship of scarce resources. This public health ethical perspective is germane to the goals and process of dementia care, public policy, and the conduct of research on human subjects.

Ethical issues do arise during the terminal stage of dementing illness, but significant ethical decisions also emerge in the everyday life of dementia caregiving. These include: (1) balancing the confidentiality of the person concerned with providing medical information; (2) the determination of decision-making capacity and engagement in a process of supported decision making as individuals experience borderline and fluctuating capacity; (3) balancing a person's previous views and values with contemporaneous best interests and well being; (4) balancing safety and freedom in the custodial care of persons with moderate or advanced dementia; (5) ethical questions of privacy arising in the use of assistive and monitoring technologies; and (6) end-of-life decision making, such as withholding and withdrawing life-prolonging treatment in the absence of specific directives or medical orders.

As emphasized by the World Health Organization, persons with dementia and their caregivers have the same human rights as every other citizen. To make this ethical ideal a reality, authorities such as the United Nations Convention on the Rights of Persons with Disabilities recognize an obligation by nation states to develop legislation, health standards and guidelines, conduct research, and provide public and professional information and education (World Health Organization, 2012).

In regard to the ethical requirements of social justice and equity, dementia care raises fundamental questions about access to high-quality care and services to support basic and functional activities of daily living. It also raises practical and political issues about how to design and fund social insurance mechanisms designed for large numbers of vulnerable people who require highly labor-intensive care for prolonged periods of time. The policy development of fair and humane care systems for people with dementia must be considered against the backdrop of extreme income inequality both in the United States and around the world. Equitable distribution of the burden of paying for needed care systems is also subject to ethical debate and cultural disagreement in regard to dementia. A broad and inclusive public process of deliberation, value identification, and priority-setting is required to address such questions as: What is a fair mix of public and private funds in an adequate and just long-term care system, populated by a disproportionate number of elderly persons afflicted with dementia? Maintaining those with dementia in the community indefinitely is very difficult; yet institutional care is expensive. Personal and family out-of-pocket expense until low-income eligibility levels for Medicaid coverage is reached, referred to as "spending down," is a typical financing pattern for dementia care today. This in turn puts pressure on state and federal funding for Medicaid programs, which are designed to serve a broad spectrum of the health needs of the poor. What is the fair share for those with dementia? How can we improve quality of life in long-term care of persons with dementia and provide appropriate medical treatments near the end of life in cost effective ways? What is the fair share of caregiving expense between families and society as a whole through a public tax system or a social insurance mechanism in which those who do not require services subsidize those who do?

Two additional high-priority ethical objectives pertain to changes in social attitudes and commitment to the values of inclusivity, non-discrimination, and mutual respect. One of these is combating the stigma that isolates and truncates the lives and opportunities of persons with dementia and their families. Strategies should be designed and implemented to improve public awareness and understanding of dementia, and to ensure that the work of caregivers is properly valued. It will also involve ensuring that dementia as a concept and people with dementia are both accepted and a visible part of society. A second ethical objective that follows from this is inclusion of people with dementia in everyday society. When possible and appropriate, persons with dementia should be supported and enabled to live in the community with access to health, social, and other support services to facilitate people leading meaningful lives in the least restrictive environments.

D. Care issues

In the clinical domain, there are many facets of innovative approaches to dementia care that need further research and exploration. The public health community should play a significant role and support innovative forms of dementia care, including design of social services and supports, along with the social and community infrastructure those improved models of care require. The different designs and approaches of dementia care all have some basic questions in common: What are the appropriate goals of care? How can comfort and safety best be integrated with promoting agency, even well into the trajectory of the illness? How should quality of life and "best interests" be understood in the context of dementia care? Are there environmental and social determinants of loss of function with dementia patients that can and should be addressed? How can we reinvent long-term care residences and environments to meet dementia care needs and sustain persons with dementia in appropriate social communities and in the human moral community? Moreover, much attention in chronic care is now focusing on community. Efforts to build age- and dementia-friendly communities raise concerns about appropriate balancing of priorities between, for example, the needs of children and elders.

E. Research issues

In the domain of research, there is a need to balance diverse and sometimes competing research interests in the investigation of dementia. Among these are the regulation and financing of translational efforts to connect research findings with clinical practices, the management and use of advances in diagnostic technologies, the active development of new models of active disease modification processes and pathways, and research on palliative care and palliative environments for persons with dementia.

There are specific ethical issues associated with human-subjects research in dementia due to the cognitive status and vulnerability of the persons necessary for these studies (Alzheimer's Association, 1997). Recruitment and availability of research subjects is also associated with the question of early diagnosis of AD, adding to these studies the implications of early diagnosis concerning risks and benefits, cost, and social and psychological consequences for persons and families.

F. Education

Health care professionals, family, friends, and other people are essential to supporting the care of persons living with dementia to provide education and service linkages that promote public health approaches. Effective communication is important to promoting an integrated model of elder-centered care and building meaningful relationships that support the health and well being of older people with dementia from ethical, legal, and educational perspectives.

Persons living with dementia should expect high-quality, accessible, equitable care from a knowledgeable, ethical, and skilled multidisciplinary team that can respond to challenges in dementia care settings. The dynamics of an integrated model will require a strong focus on education and training to prepare the multidisciplinary team to ensure best-practice principles when caring for persons with dementia to improve dementia care across settings.

The guidelines and standards originating from Alzheimer's global organizations cite a need for an educated multidisciplinary team to care for persons living with dementia to significantly improve the delivery of dementia care (Alzheimer's Association, 2013; Dementia Australia, 2017; Alzheimer's Society of Canada, 2012). Researchers have found that training and education increases the capacity to provide evidence-based best practices that improve care and reduce health disparities (Knoefel & Herman, 2015; Stanyon, Griffiths, Thomas, & Gordon, 2016; Surr, Smith, Crossland, & Robins, 2016). Developing and implementing educational strategies to support and improve the health of individuals and populations in dementia care will enhance access to care and equity.

An integrated collaborative model focusing on education may provide successful interventions to augment access and equity in dementia care settings, which would in turn support dementia care as a public health issue to address gaps in care. It is essential to train, educate, and implement a multidisciplinary framework utilizing an integrated team to ensure quality of care that will be accessible, equitable, and sustainable in the continuum of health care delivery through persons, systems, community, and populations.

V. Conclusion

The application of the phenomenological lens expands our boundaries of knowledge about suffering and enables us to locate the origin of suffering as rooted in Maternal dimensions of existence. The social ecology of suffering encompasses the social and cultural world and its environment. Large-scale population changes and refugee migrations, drought, violent weather, and political and social unrest will produce massive displacements of people from their familiar surroundings, seemingly leading to much less attentive care through the life course—for infants, children, families, undocumented immigrants and asylum seekers, and vulnerable older adults. Changes in cognitive and social health and well being, such as in the experience of dementia for older persons, is a different but equally challenging and potentially transforming type of displacement. Phenomenology suggests ways in which the Maternal Ground can be reconstituted in the face of radical disruption through social support, revitalizing agency and dignity and establishing more attentive, compassionate and palliative care to all persons as they age. Through phenomenology and a deepened understanding of subjectivity and its processes of world-constitution, the possibility looms for creatively transforming consciousness of suffering experience and intentional life in a way that may contribute to improved conditions of well being in a global ecology of suffering. The reframing of suffering as socially constituted may be fruitful in guiding the design of therapeutic approaches and the building of palliative, Maternal environments that help to mitigate suffering and enhance the flourishing of older persons through just and equitable allocation of resources, especially in this Anthropocene Period.

References

Alzheimer's Association. (1997). Protection of participants in research studies. Retrieved from: www.alz.org/documents_custom/statements/Protection_of_Participants_in _Research.pdf. Accessed December 13, 2017.

Alzheimer's Association. (2013). Alzheimer's disease facts and figures. *Alzheimer's & Dementia: Journal of the Alzheimer's Association*, 8(2), 131–168. doi: 10.1016/j .jalz.2012.02.001

Alzheimer's Disease International. (2013). *Policy brief for heads of government: The global impact of dementia 2013–2050*. London: Alzheimer's Disease International.

Alzheimer Society of Canada. (2012). A new way of looking at the impact of dementia in Canada. Retrieved from: www.alzheimer.ca/en/News-and-Events/Media-centre /Fact-sheets

Barber, M.D. (2010a). Genetic phenomenology and potentiality: A new insight into the theory of empathy in Husserl. *Análisis: Revista Colombiana de Humanidades*, 75, 61–89.

Barber, M.D. (2010b). Ethics, eidetics, and the ethical subject: A critique of Enrique Dussel's appropriation of the thought of Emmanuel Levinas. In M. Barber, L. Embree, & T. Nenon (Eds.), *Phenomenology 2010: Selected essays from North America* (pp. 355–371). Bucharest: Zeta Books.

Barber, M.D. (2011). *The intentional spectrum and intersubjectivity: Phenomenology and the Pittsburgh Neo-Hegelians*. Athens: Ohio University Press.

Barber, M.D. (2012). The cartesian residue in intersubjectivity and child development. *Schutzian Research*, *4*, 91–110.

Barber, M.D. (2013). Alfred Schutz and the problem of empathy. In L. Embree and T. Nenon (Eds.), *Husserl's Ideen* (pp. 313–326). Dordrecht, The Netherlands: Springer.

Barber, M.D. (2014). *Resistance to pragmatic tendencies in the world of working in the religious finite province of meaning*. Unpublished paper presented at Interdisciplinary Coalition of North American Phenomenologists, St. Louis, MO.

Callahan C.M., Sachs G.A., LaMantia A., Unroe, K.T., Arling, G., & Boustani, M.A. (2014). Redesigning systems of care for older adults with Alzheimer's disease. *Health Affairs*, *33*, 626–632.

Charmaz, K. (1997). *Good days, bad days: The self in chronic illness and time*. New Brunswick, NJ: Rutgers University Press.

Chin A.L., Negash, S., Hamilton, R. (2011). Diversity and disparity in dementia: The impact of ethnoracial differences in Alzheimer's disease. *Alzheimer Disease and Associated Disorders*, *25*, 187.

Cox, C. (2005). *Community care for an aging society: Issues, policies and services*. New York: Springer Publishing Company.

D'Altona S., Hunter, B., Whitehouse P.J., Brayne, C., & George, D.R. (2014). Adapting to dementia in society: A challenge for our lifetimes and a charge for public health. *Journal of Alzheimer's Disease*, *42*, 1151–1163.

Dewan, S. (2017, September 16). Saved from Harvey's floodwaters, twice: So how did she end up dead? *New York Times*. Retrieved from: www.nytimes.com/2017/09/16/us/hurricane-harvey-houston-wilma-ellis.html

Dementia Australia. (2017). Dementia statistics for Victoria. Retrieved from: www.dementia.org.au/statistics/vic

Drummond, J.J. (2002). Aristotelianism and phenomenology. In J.J. Drummond & L. Embree, *Phenomenological approaches to moral philosophy: A handbook* (pp. 15–46). Dordrecht, The Netherlands: Kluwer Academic Publishers.

Drummond, J.J. (2008a). Moral phenomenology and moral intentionality. *Phenomenology and the Cognitive Sciences*, *7*(1), 35–49.

Drummond, J.J. (2008b). The transcendental and the psychological. *Husserl Studies*, *24*, 193–204.

Embree, L. (2011). Phenomenological nursing in Schutzian perspective. In O. Wiggins & A.C. Allen (Eds.), *Clinical ethics and the necessity for stories: Essays in honor of Richard M. Zaner* (pp. 87–97). Dordrecht, The Netherlands: Springer.

Estes, C.L. (2001). *Social policy and aging: A critical perspective*. Thousand Oaks, CA: SAGE Publications.

Fentiman, L. (2003). Patient advocacy and termination from managed care organizations: Do state laws protecting health care professional advocacy make any difference? *Nebraska Law Review*, *82*(2), 508–574.

Ferreira, M.J. (2006). Misfortune of the happy: Levinas and the ethical dimensions of desire. *Journal of Religion & Ethics*, *34*(3), 461–483.

Ferreira, M.J. (2008). Kierkegaard and Levinas on four elements of the Biblical love commandment. In J.A. Simmons & D. Wood (Eds.), *Kierkegaard & Levinas: Ethics, politics & religion* (pp. 82–98). Indianapolis: Indiana University Press.

Fink, E. (1995). *Sixth Cartesian meditation: The idea of a transcendental theory of method*. (R. Bruzina, Trans.) Bloomington: Indiana University Press.

Francis, I. (2015, June 18). Laudato si. On care for our common home [Encyclical letter]. Retrieved from: http://w2.vatican.va/content/francesco/en/ encyclicals/docu ments/papa-francesco_20150524_ enciclica-laudato-si.html

Gaston, S. (2003). Levinas, disinterest and enthusiasm. *Literature and Theology, 17*(4), 407–421.

Giner-Sorolla, R. (2014). Intuition in 21st-century moral psychology. In L.M. Osbeck & B.S. Held (Eds.), *Rational intuition: Philosophical roots, scientific investigations* (pp. 338–361). New York: Cambridge University Press.

Giorgi, A. (2009). *The descriptive phenomenological method in psychology: A modified Husserlian approach.* Pittsburgh, PA: Duquesne University Press.

Husserl, E. (1970). *The crisis of European science and transcendental phenomenology.* (D. Carr, Trans.). Evanston, IL: Northwestern University Press.

Husserl, E. (1913/1989). *Ideas pertaining to a pure phenomenology and to a phenomenological philosophy. Second book: Studies in the phenomenology of constitution.* Dordrecht, The Netherlands: Springer.

Jennings, B. (2016). *Ecological governance: Toward a new social contract with the Earth.* Morgantown: West Virginia University Press.

Knoefel J., & Herman, C. (2015). Dementia care training for primary care providers: Project ECHO™ (P6.182). *Neurology, 84*(14 Supplement), P6.182.

Kolb, P. (2014). *Understanding aging and diversity: Theories and concepts.* London and New York: Routledge.

Le Couteur, D.G., Doust, J., Creasey, H., & Brayne, C. (2013). Political drive to screen for pre-dementia: Not evidence based and ignores the harms of diagnosis. *British Medical Journal, 347*, f5125.

Livingston, G., Sommerlad, A., Orgeta, V., Costafreda, S.G., Huntley, J., Ames, D., Ballard, C., Banerjee, S., Burns, A., Cohen-Mansfield, J., Cooper, C., Fox, N., Gitlin, L.N., Howard, R., Kales, H.C., Larson, E.B., Ritchie, K., Rockwood, K., Sampson, E.L., Samus, Q., Schneider, L.S., Selbæk, G., Teri, L., & Mukadam, N. (2017). Dementia prevention, intervention and care. *Lancet, 390*, 2673–2734.

Levinas, E. (1969). *Totality and infinity: An essay on exteriority.* Pittsburgh, PA: Duquesny University Press.

Levinas, E. (1981). *Otherwise than being or beyond essence.* Pittsburgh, PA: Duquesne University Press.

Marcel, G. (1949). *Being and having.* (K. Farrer, Trans.). Westminster, London: Dacre Press.

Marcel, G. (1964). *Creative fidelity.* (R. Rosthal, Trans.). New York: Farrar, Strauss & Company.

McCullough, L.B., Wilson, N.L., Rymes, J.A., & Teasdale, T. (2002). Conflicting interests: Dilemmas of decision making for patients, families, and teams. In M. Mezey, et al. (Eds.), *Ethical patient care: A casebook for geriatric health care teams* (pp. 119–135). Baltimore, MD: Johns Hopkins University Press.

Mead, G.H. (1934). *Mind, self and society.* Chicago, IL: University of Chicago Press.

Mor, V., Zinn, J., Angelleli, J., Teno, J.M., & Miller, S.C. (2004). Driven to tiers: Socioeconomic and racial disparities in the quality of nursing home care. *The Milbank Quarterly. 82*, 227–256.

Morrissey, M.B. (2011a). Phenomenology of pain and suffering: A humanistic perspective in gerontological health and social work. *Journal of Social Work in End-of Life and Palliative Care, 7*(1), 14–38.

Morrissey, M.B. (2011b). *Suffering and decision making among seriously ill elderly women.* Unpublished dissertation, Fordham University.

Morrissey, M.B. (2011c). Expanding consciousness of suffering at the end of life: An ethical and gerontological response in palliative social work. *Schutzian Research*, 3, 77–104.

Morrissey, M.B. (2015a). *Suffering narratives of older adults.* London and New York: Routledge.

Morrissey, M.B. (2015b, August). *Toward a transcendentally informed phenomenology of suffering: Humanizing suffering—The task for psychology.* Paper presented at the American Psychological Association Convention, Toronto, Canada.

Morrissey, M.B., & Barber, M. (2014). Phenomenology. In B. Jennings (Ed.), *Bioethics* (4th ed.). Farmington Hills, MI: Macmillan Reference USA.

Morrissey, M.B., & Whitehouse, P. (2016). From suffering to holistic flourishing: Emancipatory maternal care practices—A substantive notion of the good. *Journal of Theoretical and Philosophical Psychology, 36*(2),115–127.

Morrissey, M.B. (2016, May). *Contributions of transcendental theory of method to understanding of suffering and maternal analogy.* Paper presented at Interdisciplinary Coalition of North American Phenomenologists VIII, Phoenix, Arizona.

Morrissey, M.B. (2018). Suffering in the Anthropocene Era: Contributions of phenomenology to understanding the world-constituting role of subjectivity. In: D.A. DellaSala, and M.I. Goldstein (Eds.), *The encyclopedia of the Anthropocene, Vol. 4,* (pp. 147–150). Oxford: Elsevier.

National Institutes of Health. (2013). *The dementias: Hope through research.* NIH Publication No. 13-2252. Retrieved from: https://catalog.ninds.nih.gov/pubstatic //17-NS-2252/17-NS-2252.pdf

Reisner, N., Fink, S., & Yee, V. (2017, September 13). Eight dead from sweltering nursing home as Florida struggles after Irma. *New York Times.* Retrieved from: www .nytimes.com/2017/09/13/us/nursing-home-deaths-florida.html

Schutz, A. (1957/2010). Das Problem der transzendentalen Intersubjektivität bei Husserl, 5, 81–107 (The problem of transcendental intersubjectivity in Husserl, Studies in Phenomenological Philosophy, 51–91). A recent translation with comments by Dorion Cairns (Trans.). *Schutzian Research, 2,* 9–52.

Schutz, A. (1996). *Collected papers, Vol. IV.* H. Wagner, G. Psathas, & F. Kersten (Eds.). Dordrecht, The Netherlands: Kluwer Academic Publishers.

Stanyon, M.R., Griffiths, A., Thomas, S.A., & Gordon, A.L. (2016). The facilitators of communication with people with dementia in a care setting: An interview study with healthcare workers. *Age and Ageing, 45*: 164–170.

Surr C.A., Smith S.J., Crossland J., & Robins, J. (2016). Impact of a person-centered dementia care training programme on hospital staff attitudes, role efficacy and perceptions of caring for people with dementia: A repeated measures study. *International Journal of Nursing Studies, 53,* 144–151.

Turkewitz, J., & Medina, J. (2017, September 1). For vulnerable older adults, a harrowing sense of being trapped. *New York Times.* Retrieved from: www.nytimes .com/2017/09/01/us/storm-elderly-harvey.html

UK Health Forum. (2014). Blackfriars consensus on promoting brain health: Reducing risks for dementia in the population. Retrieved January 12, 2016 from: http://nhfshare.heartforum.org.uk/RMAssets/Reports/Blackfriars%20consen sus%20%20_V18.pdf

Wertz, F.J. (1981). The birth of the infant: A developmental perspective. *Journal of Phenomenological Psychology, 12*(1), 205–220.

Wertz, F.J. (2005). Phenomenological research methods for counseling psychology. *Journal of Counseling Psychology, 52*(2), 167–177.

Wertz, F.J. (2010). The method of eidetic analysis for psychology. In T. Cloonan & C. Thiboutot (Eds.), *The redirection of psychology: Essays in honor of Amedeo P. Giorgi,* (pp. 261–278). Montreal, Quebec: Le Cercle Interdisciplinaire de Recherches Phénoménologiques (CIRP), l'Université du Québec.

Wertz, F.J., Charmaz, K., McMullen, L.M., Josselson, R., Anderson, R., & McSpadden, E. (2011). *Five ways of doing qualitative analysis: Phenomenological psychology, grounded theory, discourse analysis, narrative research and intuitive inquire.* New York: Guilford Press.

Wertz, F.J. (2016). Outline of the relationship among transcendental phenomenology, phenomenological psychology and sciences of persons. *Schutzian Research, 8,* 139–162.

Westphal, M. (2008). *Levinas and Kierkegaard in dialogue.* Indianapolis: Indiana University Press.

Whitehouse P.J., & George D.R. (2015). A tale of two reports: What recent publications from the Alzheimer's Association and Institute of Medicine say about the state of the field. *Journal of Alzheimer's Disease, 49*: 21–25.

World Health Organization (WHO). (2012). *Dementia: A public health priority.* Geneva, Switzerland. Retrieved from:www.who.int/mental_health/publications/dementia_report_educatio2012/en/

Zaner, R. (2002). Making music together while growing older: Further reflections on intersubjectivity. *Human Studies* 25: 1–18, 2002. © 2002 Kluwer Academic Publishers. Printed in the Netherlands.

Bibliography

McCullough, L.B., Wilson, N.L., Teasdale, T.A., Kolpakchi, A.L., & Skelly, J.R. (1993). Mapping personal, familial, and professional values in long term care decisions. *Gerontologist, 33*(3), 324–332.

Picasso, P. (1937). *Guernica.* [Painting.] Retrieved January 31, 2017 from: www.museo reinasofia.es/coleccion/obra/ guernica

Part Two

Paradigm shifts in delivery systems and financing

3   Moving from fragmentation to integrated, community-based services

I.   Introduction: Long-term services and supports

Providing care for older adults requires a broad range of services to allow chronically disabled people to participate in everyday activities. Even those who are not chronically disabled need support to help them remain in their homes as they age. Broadly speaking, no coordinated system of long-term services and supports (LTSS) exists that can incorporate both medical and non-medical "wraparound" social services to address all daily living needs. With some exceptions, which will be explored in later chapters, no set "formal system" enables access to these services, especially for those who are considered middle class; the costs exceed most people's ability to pay. The future of aging care relies on the reconfiguration of services to create a seamless network with comprehensive service models (Reinhard, Kassner, Houser, & Mollica, 2011). While legislation does reflect a shift toward increasing care for older adults, limitations remain in the current ad hoc, "patchwork quilt" structure. Most government funding was conceived as a supplement to other programs, leaving a gap that often places eldercare responsibilities primarily on families. Our health care system relies heavily on this family support, as limitations in funding often create the need for additional out-of-pocket supports and services. Examining these shifts and historical implications reveals a fragmented pattern with deep historical roots.

Almshouses, which operated from the late seventeenth century to the early twentieth century based on a model imported from Britain, provide important context for our understanding of institutional care. These "poorhouses" dispensed food, shelter, and medical care, but left residents stigmatized and unable to lead independent lives (Achenbaum & Carr, 2014). Almshouses were widely criticized after the turn of the twentieth century for low standards of care that led to poor health and poor quality of life among their residents. Until the Social Security Act of 1935, programs available to help financially limited older Americans were deeply limited. While this particular practice of institutionalizing the poor was eventually ended, the Hill-Burton Act (1954), which gave rise to the nursing-home industry for older adults in need of skilled nursing care, ended up replicating some of those earlier conditions.

The Hill-Burton Act provided federal grants for nursing homes built in conjunction with hospitals. Funding declined in the early 1970s, coinciding with national scandals that exposed abuses in nursing homes and other care institutions, which bore similarities to almshouses where people had felt forced to spend their final days confined to poor conditions.

Today, advocates for health care overwhelmingly agree that affordable access to long-term services and supports (LTSS) is critical for our aging population. Yet most Americans lack any insurance to cover the costs of these services. As the United States does not have a single, unified system, public policy plays a significant role in shaping long-term services and supports by establishing eligibility frameworks, the scope of benefits, and the structure and financing of delivery systems. The prohibitive cost of services for most middle-income families makes public policy critically important. Over the years, policy makers have explored ways to drive diversion from institutional settings by supporting structures that strengthen community-based supports and maximize independence. While today there is heightened recognition of what some call a "graying America," in fact life expectancy has been increasing for many years, and concerns about meeting the needs of the growing population of older adults have been on policy agendas for decades (Sade, 2012).

II.   Medicare and Medicaid

Medicare and Medicaid, both enacted in 1965, have provisions aimed at meeting the needs of older adults, but come with specific rules about which services are covered, duration of benefits, eligibility, and out-of-pocket costs. Federal legislation and regulations, and their many different state and local interpretations, all contribute to a complicated long-term care delivery environment. Medicare pays for people aged 65 and older who also qualify for Social Security benefits, people under age 65 with certain disabilities, and anyone with end-stage renal disease (kidney disease requiring dialysis or a transplant). It covers medically necessary care that includes both acute care, like doctors' visits, prescription drugs, and hospital stays, and short-term services. It will help pay for short stays in a skilled nursing facility, hospice care, and, in certain cases, a portion of the costs of home health care. However, Medicare does not pay for personal care, such as bathing and dressing or custodial care (Centers for Medicare & Medicaid Services, 2017). Medicaid helps people with limited resources pay for some or all of their health care needs. Unlike Medicare, Medicaid does pay for custodial care in nursing homes and at home. Rules governing eligibility and covered services are based on federal requirements that allow each state to choose its own criteria, including maximum thresholds for income and assets.

The biggest difference between Medicare and Medicaid relates to long-term planning; the latter covers nursing-home care, while the former does not. Today, in the absence of any other public program covering long-term care, Medicaid has become the default provider of long-term care services for those with limited income. This leaves middle-class Americans with complex decisions as to how to pay for their long-term care needs, with many surprised to learn that Medicare, which exists in large part to serve older populations, nevertheless does not cover most of these costs. In fact, when Medicare was enacted it was likely designed to work in conjunction with other legislation, such as the Older Americans Act (OAA) passed the same year, not as a catch-all for the health needs of older middle-class people.

A. Older Americans Act (OAA)

The Older Americans Act (1965) was passed in response to concerns over the lack of community-based supports for older adults. Under the OAA, all individuals aged 60 and older are eligible for community-based services, with specific attention given to low-income and minority older people. The legislation provided states with grants to coordinate community-planning and social services, research-and-development projects, and personnel training in the field of aging. The law also established the Administration on Aging, which later created the Administration on Community Living, to administer programs and serve as a focal resource (O'Shaughnessy, 2004).

The OAA was envisioned as a means to create positive momentum regarding long-term care opportunities for the growing elderly population (Parikh, Montgomery, & Lynn, 2015). In 1965, many older Americans lacked health insurance, and few retirement plans provided this type of coverage. There are no mandatory fees for services within the OAA's grant programs, and volunteers play a critical role in the delivery of services.

In comparison to Medicare and Medicaid, which permanently altered the American health landscape, the OAA was considered a less significant reform. Although its scope is limited relative to the large numbers of older adults, the infrastructure it established remains a vital entry point for providing needed resources to this population. The OAA plays a key role in the delivery of social and nutrition services to older Americans and their caregivers, authorizing a broad array of service programs through a national network of Area Agencies on Aging (AAA). However, the funding for these programs has not kept pace with the growing aging population and the significant challenges they face, leaving a gaping hole in available support for older Americans, especially those who are middle class (Parikh et al., 2015).

The realization that adding community-based supports could enable a greater number of older adults to "age in place," rather than enter institutionalized settings, prompted exploration by policy makers. Since Medicaid has long played a vital role in providing long-term care, the federal insurance program was at the forefront of testing stronger community-based supports that maximize independence and divert the need for institutional care. In the early 1980s, the recognition that a disproportionate percentage of Medicaid resources were being used for institutional long-term care spurred several studies offering financial arguments for community-based care over institutionalization. Additional research indicated that one-third of Medicaid-eligible persons residing in nursing facilities would likely be able to remain in the community with moderate levels of additional support. This unnecessary use of institutional care, described as an "institutional bias" within the Medicaid structure, was accompanied by reports that residents in skilled nursing facilities were not satisfied with the quality of life. These preferences, and the prohibitive costs of such care, led to several changes being made towards encouraging a more community-based paradigm.

B.   HCBS waiver programs

Medicaid long-term care services are usually distributed through a state plan or home and community-based services (HCBS) waiver. States submit a plan describing which groups are eligible and which services are covered. Once approved, these services must be available statewide and offered to all Medicaid enrollees who qualify. Since home and community-based care is attractive to those in need of LTSS, and may have cost-saving potential, several states have tested possibilities for spending more of their LTSS-focused funding on these types of services rather than institutional care (Tritz, 2005).

The home and community-based services (HCBS) waiver program is Medicaid's vehicle for providing long-term care services in community-based settings. Established through Section 2176 of the Omnibus Budget Reconciliation Act of 1981, it was also incorporated into the Social Security Act at Section 1915(c). Because of this critical step, many individuals who might have been institutionalized instead received the support they needed to remain in their homes, and at a cost no higher than institutional care (Duckett, 2000).

The HCBS waiver program allows states the flexibility to offer a range of services that Medicaid would not otherwise cover, such as case management, personal care, home health aides, adult day and habilitation programs, and respite care. Medicaid can also approve additional services for waiver participants to avoid institutionalization if cost-effective, such as transportation, in-home support services, meals, communication and home modifications, and adult day care. Individuals with physical or developmental disabilities and people who have mental illness can also receive waiver programs in addition to older adults. The Health Care Financing Administration (HCFA) reviews each waiver, but states have flexibility in designing their own programs, allowing for creativity in developing alternatives to institutionalization. This flexibility has resulted in a great deal of diversity among HCBS waiver program benefits, both across the country and within individual states. The waiver has enabled programs initially funded exclusively with state or local dollars to tap into the state-federal matching and reimbursement structure (Shirk, 2006).

The Deficit Reduction Act (DRA) of 2005 made it easier to qualify for HCBS by adding an option for states to offer it without a waiver under the Medicaid state plan, which allowed states to develop different functional eligibility definitions for institutional care and for home- and community-based care. Importantly, this change also allowed states to continue to limit the number of HCBS participants, but without having to apply for waiver renewals or demonstrate cost-neutrality (Shirk, 2006).

Through the 1115 waiver program—so named because of its origins in Section 1115 of the Social Security Act—states can design consumer-directed, long-term care programs and directly pay beneficiaries or their representatives. Consumer-directed services can give individuals with disabilities the authority to determine the services they need and flexibility to manage them within a pre-defined budget (Tritz, 2005). The Centers for Medicare & Medicaid Services (CMS), along with other organizations, have developed initiatives to facilitate these programs.

III. Newer legislation and initiatives

A. Americans with Disabilities Act

The judicial system plays an influential role in influencing long-term care policy. In the 1980s, a series of class action lawsuits revealed civil rights violations of individuals with developmental disabilities living in state institutions. A formal advocacy movement, organized by parents and disability advocates on behalf of the developmentally disabled, shifted the momentum in the direction of community-based residences and supports. The Americans with Disabilities Act (ADA) enacted in 1990 represented a sea of change for waiver programs. The federal regulations required that states provide services, "in the most integrated setting appropriate to the needs of qualified individuals ... rather than in institutions" (28 CFR § 35.130[d]). Court rulings thus began to uphold the rights of people with disabilities to receive care in the community. The most notable case, *Olmstead v. L.C.* (1999), upheld the right to receive treatment in community settings if such placement is appropriate, not opposed by the individual, and can be accommodated with available resources. In addition, the U.S. Supreme Court found in the Olmstead ruling that institutionalization severely limits a person's quality of life, including interaction with family and friends and ability to work—an important affirmation of community-based, long-term care (527 U.S. 581 [1999]). Under the ADA, states can comply with the requirement to make reasonable accommodations to avoid discrimination based on disability in part by demonstrating their plans for placing people with disabilities in less restrictive settings, such as waiting lists that move at a reasonable pace. Following the Olmstead decision, the federal government emphasized moving people from institutions to communities and developed steps for state Medicaid directors to ensure compliance. In particular, HCBS waivers have served as a valuable tool to help states build infrastructure for integrated home- and community-based services.

While these policy changes helped Medicaid shed its bias toward institutional settings, the infrastructure they helped create is not fully equipped to meet the challenges associated with healthy aging. Successful aging relies on the intersection of multiple sectors that include housing, financial support, health, and social services. Older Americans need professionals who are trained to provide long-term care, yet shortages and barriers to necessary education among such workers remain. Furthermore, with systems and supports that are often piecemeal, there is no effective means to adequately evaluate the quality of care.

The *State Long-Term Services and Supports Scorecard*, first published in 2011 and updated with a follow-up report in 2014, measures state-level performance of LTSS systems using a multidimensional approach (Reinhard et al., 2011). The second edition measures LTSS system performance across five key dimensions: affordability and access, patients' level of choice, quality of life and care, support for family caregivers, and effective transitions. The report notes that in most states the cost of nursing home care exceeds the median income of older Americans and finds wide variation across all dimensions of state LTSS system performance. The states with the most success in providing quality health care accessibly, it contends, are the ones where public policy has played an integral role in creating that health care climate (Reinhard et al., 2011).

B.   Affordable Care Act

The Affordable Care Act (ACA), passed in 2010 under President Obama's administration, with the aim of making health insurance more affordable and accessible, provided incentives for states to improve access to community-based long-term supports (Kaiser Family Foundation, 2011):

- The State Balancing Incentive Program, under the ACA, provided enhanced federal matching payments (FMAP) to eligible states that made specified structural program changes. Effective in 2011 were the following measures: establish a statewide system of single entry points for LTSS; adopt certain case management practices; and develop and use standard assessment tools in a uniform manner across the state.
- The Money Follows the Person demonstration was extended through 2016. Established in 2007, the demonstration allowed states to help residents of institutions transition to the community by providing a range of services including transition, housing, and technological assistance. States received an enhanced federal match rate (75–90% FMAP) for each person who successfully transitions to the community from nursing homes. The new requirements also reduced the institutional length of stay needed to qualify for benefits from six months to 90 days.
- The 1915(i) Home and Community-Based Services state plan option established in the 2005 Deficit Reduction Act (DRA) has been available to states since January 2007, but only a small number use it. Under the option, individuals do not have to qualify for an institutional level of care to be eligible for community-based services. The ACA allowed states to

broaden the eligibility criteria. Benefits must be available state wide and states cannot place caps on enrollment, but services may be targeted to specific populations.

- The Community First Choice Option created a new state plan option in 2011 that covered a broad range of services and supports, including benefits such as one month's rent, utility deposits, or household furnishings, for Medicaid-eligible consumers who require an institutional level of care.
- The ACA appropriated $10 million per year from 2010 to 2014 to expand Aging and Disability Resource Centers for the purposing of serving as community access points for persons seeking LTSS.

While no consensus exists on the definition of "middle class," the median household income in America was $59,039 in 2016, according to Sept. 2017 census reports. The Pew Research Center categorizes middle class as people with an income between two-thirds and double the national median. As only 6.1% of people earn household incomes above $200,000 per year, according to the census, most Americans do not have the financial resources to pay for the substantial out-of-pocket costs to cover the cost of LTSS. The Census Bureau estimated that 41.5% of American households earned between $35,000 and $100,000 annually in 2015. Given that neither Medicare nor Medicaid is designed to help middle-income Americans in need of long-term care, older individuals often turn to family members or forgo the full breadth of services that they may need. Ultimately, they may come to rely on services offered by their states, but middle-income people can only access those community programs by spending down and impoverishing themselves to meet eligibility requirements. In later chapters, we explore the growth of movements to provide services that will not exclude the middle class, a necessity within a system providing few supports for individuals with moderate means.

The initial legislation for the ACA included provisions to increase access to LTSS for older Americans who would not qualify for Medicaid, but this piece did not make it into the final legislation. The CLASS Act (Community Living Assistance Services and Supports) would have established a voluntary insurance program requiring individuals to pay premiums to participate. The CLASS Act was the first national, non-means-tested program focusing exclusively on long-term care. Rather than pay for 24-hour care, the policy would have supplemented community supports that enable individuals to avoid or delay admission to nursing homes. Although the cost of the CLASS program was relatively small compared to Medicaid or Medicare, it could have covered significant costs of home and community-based services, offsetting a portion of institutional costs. The demise of CLASS, the only provision truly aimed at assisting middle-income individuals with long-term care, represented a lost opportunity to health care reformers for changing the direction of long-term care policy and decreasing the burden on Medicaid. Despite the CLASS Act's failure to become law, advocates saw its introduction as a statement of recognition by the U.S. government that long-term care is a major policy concern, which will eventually need to be addressed. The benefits and cost-saving potential of community-based supports to facilitate aging in place mean that leaders in health care will likely continue to explore new avenues to make such services more accessible.

IV.   Economic and social arguments for aging in place

Prior to the Affordable Care Act, approximately 40 million Americans lacked medical insurance. Even today, more than 200 million Americans lack any insurance protection against the costs of long-term services and supports designed to assist older adults with disabilities in performing activities of daily living, from bathing to household chores. This assistance is critical for people whose physical, cognitive, or chronic conditions prevent them from performing instrumental activities of daily living on their own for an extended period, typically 90 days or more (Reinhard et al., 2011).

For many older adults, aging well requires a coordinated system of supports and services addressing that address all daily living needs. Adequate LTSS requires integration across a range of health care services and settings, including family involvement, especially where this provides respite to relatives who have become providers and decision-makers (Lynn, 2016). Reports from AARP consistently reveal that over 90% of older adults wish to stay in their homes, but many are likely to live alone while handling chronic conditions (Harrell, Lynott, Guzman, & Lampkin, 2014). The concept of "aging in place" or "aging in community" as an alternative to institutional care has grown significantly in popularity over the last several years. More individuals deemed chronically disabled need care and assistance, both inside and outside the health care sector, yet payment and caregiving constraints remain unfortunate realities.

Depending on the economic level of the individual, people may be living in homes exposed to various environmental and situational challenges that lead to inadequate/unsanitary living conditions (e.g., poor indoor air quality, cigarette smoke, chemicals, poorly maintained housing). Home hygiene and methods of preventing infections may be at a reduced level and could contribute to the individual's need to be institutionalized. Many of these circumstances can be corrected through educating individuals and/or their family members and with vigilance from support personnel who may have access to the home (e.g., volunteers, public health nurses, environmental health personnel). The individual and family frequently can be taught appropriate techniques for improved living conditions (Koren, 2017).

Overcoming the barriers of decreased functional capacity is critical to the goal of maintaining independence. With moderate levels of support and formalized coordinated efforts, such as social services, older adults may delay or avoid nursing home admission. Several forces over the past few decades have brought consensus within health policy discourse that aging-in-place models are economically as well as socially beneficial. Aging in place provides a higher quality of life for older Americans who wish to remain in their communities, without the excessive cost of institutionalization. Yet without proper supports, aging-in-place may lead to unmet needs, social isolation, inadequate health care, physical and emotional vulnerability, and ultimately institutionalization.

As mentioned, the current system can sometimes force people in need of nursing home services to "spend down" their assets to qualify for these services, which they can obtain only through Medicaid, not Medicare. Over the years, studies evaluating the cost-effectiveness of Medicaid HCBS have shown lower average costs per individual for home-based care compared to institutional care. Overall, these community-based alternatives are less expensive than traditional institutionalized care, although individual expenditures for these services continue to rise as they are expanded and grow in popularity (Marek, Stetzer, Adams, Popejoy, & Rantz, 2012).

Viewing care for the aging through a purely medical lens neglects other factors crucial to determining whether older adults can maintain independence and quality of life. The concept of "patient-centered care" grew out of a recognition that individuals require a coordination of sectors that go beyond the medical realm. However, the use of this phrase often comes across as an advertisement strategy designed to address negative preconceptions of health care's "disease-based" or "silo-driven" elements, rather than a true paradigm shift. Indeed, even the term "patient-centered care," while shifting focus to the individual, still places that individual within a medical framework by identifying people as patients first and foremost. Care that is truly person-centered requires not only this medical model, but a social model encompassing all aspects of a person's life and well being. The first step in that process is making the importance of a social model to successful aging more widely understood; only after that can the long, arduous discussions begin about how best to insert that model.

A social model for aging encompasses any services or supports that let individuals maintain their independence, from help with home maintenance to assistance with activities of daily living such as bathing, dressing, and eating. Crucially, it also involves taking steps to reduce social isolation and enabling a person to participate in meaningful activities. Supports go beyond just services to include assistive devices, such as wheelchairs, and home modifications intended to help seniors remain in their homes (O'Neill, Wilson, & Morrow-Howell, 2010).

Gerontologists have long maintained that staying actively engaged in civic life is correlated with successful aging and overall well being. Social relationships, a fundamental part of active engagement, can have a profound effect on not just well being, but long-term morbidity and mortality (Holt-Lunstad, Smith, & Layton, 2010). These relationships are forged and strengthened through activities that bring older adults together, including recreation, faith-based endeavors, and volunteering. A 2009 meta-analysis from A 2009 study examined cumulative empirical evidence across 148 independent studies, looking through data from 308,849 individuals followed for an average of 7.5 years. The study revealed that "individuals with adequate social relationships have a 50% greater likelihood of survival compared to those with poor or insufficient social relationships." These results remained consistent across several factors, including age, sex, initial health status, follow-up period, and cause of death, suggesting that the association between social relationships and mortality may be generalized, a finding that has groundbreaking implications (Holt-Lunstad et al., 2010).

Experts in the field of aging largely agree that the more people can do for themselves, the greater their overall self-esteem and satisfaction. Having opportunities to help others through structured volunteering and civic engagement can bring even greater satisfaction. Several private, public, and nonprofit organizations work to provide opportunities for lifelong learning, volunteering and public service, and advocacy for older Americans, such as the American Society on Aging, Gerontological Society of America, and National Council on Aging (O'Neill et al., 2010).

The concept of aging in place continues to present an attractive option for policy makers and individuals alike, given its numerous financial and social benefits. As concerns magnify over the challenge of providing sufficient aging services for Baby Boomers—the largest increase among older Americans in history—the need for policies that encourage community-based supports and services will only grow in urgency.

V.   Hospice as a model

As we have established, appropriate care for older adults requires a broad range of services if we are to help chronically disabled people perform everyday activities. Crucially, however, people not considered chronically disabled also require support to remain in their homes as they age. In the twenty-first century, health policy has explored ways to drive diversion from institutional settings by strengthening community-based supports, but the long-term care environment remains quite fragmented overall.

The integration of social and health-related services through transitions among different settings and environments is therefore critical. A number of community-based models and innovations aimed at improving quality support for older adults offer great promise for coordinating such transitions. Several of these initiatives, explored in later chapters, attempt to address the needs of older Americans through a combination of traditional government services, demonstration projects and pilot programs, or community-based nonprofits. These models must be able to integrate palliative and end-of-life options for older adults as their needs change through the aging process. The successes of the hospice movement, an end-of-life care model introduced in the United States in the 1970s, can provide valuable insight into the policy challenges associated with the paradigm shift on delivery of care.

Hospice professionals have long known that true patient-centered care requires an interdisciplinary approach that fully takes into account patients and their families. Similarly, patient-centered care demands case management to assist with transitions between settings—whether hospital, skilled nursing facility, in-patient hospice units, or the home—as the patient progresses in their illness trajectory. The interdisciplinary team helps in managing all aspects of care, including the respite and psychosocial services for family members who have become a part of the larger "unit of care." Being able to offer flexible levels of support and provide for the well being of patients and families through these transitions represents a critical component of good hospice care. Even so, hospice care did not immediately find widespread support in the United States. It took time for the medical establishment to broadly accept its philosophy; in the meantime, advocates had to make a case for reimbursement under Medicare and Medicaid. While hospice's redeeming qualities in terms of fostering positive experiences for patients and families have earned the movement great esteem, the attraction to policy makers lay in its potential for cutting costs. The prospect of these savings in our health care system, under the banner of "good deaths," eventually provided arguments in favor of hospice care that were too compelling for policy makers to ignore.

VI.   Conclusion

Forging partnerships toward a coordinated "aging in community" platform is critical to promoting change. Anyone familiar with the advocacy movement for people with developmental disabilities knows that it was parents and siblings visiting Washington, DC and marching to state capitols, armed with pictures and stories of their loved ones, who were far too compelling to ignore. These parents often describe realizing from the day their children were born that they were now advocates, and that the system for supporting these individuals needed to change. As a society, we view the needs of our aging population as reflecting a natural progression of the lifespan. The lack of coordination or necessary funding to meet this demand is not necessarily viewed as an omission, or lack of attention. However, if all informal caregivers marched to state capitols with pictures of their loved ones, expressing worries about mom or dad falling, the prohibitive cost of assisted living or skilled nursing, and the opportunity cost of informal care, the reinvigoration of our aging infrastructure would become paramount.

References

Achenbaum, A., & Carr, L.C. (2014, July 21). A brief history of aging services in the United States. Retrieved from: www.asaging.org/blog/brief-history-aging-services -united-states

Americans with Disabilities Act of 1990, 28 CFR § 35.130[d]). (1990).

Americans with Disabilities Act of 1990. Pub L. 101–336, 104 Stat. 327.

Atkins, S., Cote, S., & Houten, P. (2010). How boomers can help improve health care—Emerging encore career opportunities in health care. *Civic ventures.* Retrieved from: www.metlife.com/assets/cao/foundation/JobsHealthPaper3-5-10.pdf

Burwell, B., Sredl, K., & Eiken, S. (2009, December). *Medicaid long-term care expenditures FY 2008.* Cambridge, MA: Thomson Reuters.

Centers for Medicare & Medicaid Services. (2005, Winter). Key milestones in Medicare and Medicaid history, selected years: 1965–2003. *Health Care Financing Review, 27*(2), 1.

Committee for a Responsible Federal Budget. (2011). Summary table of fiscal plans. Retrieved from: www.crfb.org/sites/default/files/CRFB_Summary_Table_of_Fiscal _Plans.pdf

Congressional Budget Office. (1997, March). Reducing the deficit: Spending and revenue options. Retrieved from: www.cbo.gov/sites/default/files/cbofiles/ftpdocs/0xx /doc6/doc06.pdf

Dentzer, S. (2011). Innovation: Needed, but not rocket science. *Health Affairs, 30*(3), 378.

Deficit Reduction Act. (2005). Pub L. 109–171, 120 Stat. 4.

Duckett, M.J., & Guy, M. (2000). Home and community-based services waivers. *Health Care Financing Review, 22*(1), 123–125.

Grabowski, D. (2006). The cost-effectiveness of non-institutional long-term care services: Review and synthesis of the most recent evidence. *Medical Care Research and Review, 63*(1), 3–28.

Harrell, R., Lynott, J., Guzman, S., & Lamkin, C. (2014, April). What is livable? Community preference of older adults. Retrieved from: www.aarp.org/ppi/issues livable-communities/info-2015/what-is-livable-AARP-ppi-liv-com.html

Holt-Lunstad, J., Smith, T., & Layton, J. (2010). Social relationships and mortality risk: A meta-analytic review. *PLoS Medicine, 7*(7). https://doi.org/10.1371/journal .pmed.1000316

Hill-Burton Act of 1954. Pub L. 79–725, 60 Stat. 1040.

Johnson, K., & Wilson, K. (2010). Current economic status of older adults in the United States: A demographic analysis. Retrieved from: www.ncoa.org/assets/files /pdf/Economic-Security-Trends-for-Older-Adults-65-and-Older-March-2010.pdf

Justice, D. (2010, April). Long-term services and supports and chronic care coordination: Policy advances enacted by the Patient Protection and Affordable Care Act [Brief]. Retrieved from: www.nashp.org/long-term-services-and-supports-and -chronic-care-coordination-policy-advances-enacted/

Kaiser Commission on Medicaid and the Uninsured. (2011, February). A challenge for states: Assuring timely access to optimal long-term services and supports in the community [Brief]. Retrieved from: www.kff.org/health-reform /issue-brief/a-challenge-for-states-assuring-timely-access/

Koren, H. (2017). *Best practices for environmental health: Environmental pollution, protection, quality and sustainability.* New York and London: Routledge.

Lynn, J. (2016). *MediCaring communities: Getting what we want and need in frail old age at an affordable cost.* CreateSpace Publishers.

Marek, K., Stetzer, F., Adams, S., Popejoy, L., & Rantz, M. (2012). Aging in place versus nursing home care: Comparison of costs to Medicare and Medicaid. *Research in Gerontological Nursing, 5*(2), 123–129. doi: 10.3928/19404921-20110802-01

O'Neill, G., Wilson, S.F., & Morrow-Howell, N. (2010). The civic enterprise: Advancing civic engagement opportunities in later life. In G. O'Neill, & S.F. Wilson (Eds.), *Civic engagement in an older America* (pp. 1–5). Washington, DC: Gerontological Society of America.

O'Shaughnessy, C. (2004). *Older Americans Act: History of appropriations, FY1966–FY2004* [Government report]. Washington, DC: Congressional Research Service.

O'Shaughnessy, C., Stone, J., Thomas, G., & Shrestha. L.B. (2007, March 15). *Long-term care: Consumers, providers and payers* [Government report]. Washington, DC: Congressional Research Service.

Older Americans Act of 1965. Pub. L. 89–73, 79 Stat. 218.

Olmstead v. L.C., 527 U.S. 581 (1999).

Omnibus Budget Reconciliation Act of 1981. Pub L. 97–35, 95 Stat. 357.

Parikh, R.B., Montgomery, A., & Lynn, J. (2015). The Older Americans Act at 50—Community-based care in a value driven era. *New England Journal of Medicine, 373*(5), 399–401.

Pew Research Center. (2016, May 11). America's shrinking middle class: A close look at changes within metropolitan areas. Retrieved from: www.pewsocialtrends .org/2016/05/11/americas-shrinking-middle-class-a-close-look-at-changes-within -metropolitan-areas/

Reinhard, S.C., Kassner, E., Houser, A, & Mollica, R. (2011, September). Raising expectations: A state scorecard on long-term services and supports for older adults, people with physical disabilities, and family caregivers. Retrieved from: https:// assets.aarp.org/rgcenter/ppi/ltc/ltss_scorecard.pdf

Sade, R.M. (2012). Introduction: The graying of America: Challenges and controversies. *Journal of Law, Medicine & Ethics, 40*: 6–9. doi:10.1111/j.1748-720X.2012.00639.x

Semega, J.L., Fontenot, K.R., & Kollar, M.A. (2017). Income and poverty in the United States: 2016. Retrieved from: www.census.gov/content/dam/Census/library /publications/2017/demo/P60-259.pdf

Shirk, C. (2006). *Rebalancing long-term care: The role of the Medicaid HCBS Waiver Program*. Washington, DC: National Health Policy Forum.

Social Security Act of 1935. Pub L. 74–271, 49 Stat. 620.

The Patient Protection and Affordable Care Act. (2010) Pub L. 111–148, 124 Stat. 119.

Tritz, K. (2005). *Long-term care: Consumer-directed services under Medicaid. CRS Report for Congress*. Washington, DC: Congressional Research Service.

Wright, B. (2005). Direct care workers in long-term care. Retrieved from: https://assets .aarp.org/rgcenter/il/dd117_workers.pdf

4   Development of elder-centered systems of care

I.   Introduction: Importance of delivery systems

The elderly form the most complicated demographic and patient population in the health care system. For the most part, younger patients are healthy, with either occasional, self-limited acute illnesses, which resolve themselves fairly simply, or a single chronic illness to be managed. With more than two-thirds of people over 65 having multiple diagnoses and 40% taking multiple medications, this group includes the highest utilizers of the system, with costs approximately four times higher than the average person. Although people over 65 account for only 13% of the population, they account for 34% of prescriptions and OTC use (Institute of Medicine, 2008). As care becomes more complex during the aging process, the need for interdisciplinary and inter-professional collaboration becomes more critical. More than any other population, the elderly are vulnerable to systemic gaps in health care and infrastructure on which the quality of their care depends.

Before the 1940s and 1950s, medicine in the United States was largely a decentralized cottage industry centered on individual physician practices, mostly comprised of local general practitioners. At this time, medical knowledge and capacities were simpler, with limited diagnostics and therapeutics. Health care insurance—public or private—was almost non-existent (American College of Health Executives, 2007). Care options and funding sources were limited, consigning most care to take place in the home, with only limited use of hospitals and specialists. Advances in medical knowledge drove the shift toward hospital-centric, specialty-based medicine that incorporated multiple practitioners with differing areas of specialization into a patient's care, thus reducing the role of the primary family physician. Between 1960 and 2010, the percentage of primary care physicians in the physician workforce declined 17% from 50% to 33%, while specialty care training programs grew by more than 30% (Committee on the Governance and Financing of Graduate Medical Education, 2014). The development of government-based health insurance via Medicare and Medicaid, along with the advent of employer-based commercial health insurance, supported and reinforced this trend toward specialization, as did labor movements during this period.

For decades, the U.S. health care system remained fragmented, despite a need for changes that would reflect the increased complexity of care brought on by medical progress. This model sufficed for younger patients who were in good health or had less complex isolated chronic illnesses. The inelastic economic model for the health care system, in which government or employers shoulder costs for the majority of policies, shielded individuals from the cost of care while giving purchasers little incentive to prioritize quality of services, buffering the typical competitive drivers that prompt structural changes in other industries (Ringel, Hosek, Vollaard, & Mahnovskiet, 2002). The incipient health maintenance organization (HMO) movement in the eighties and early nineties signaled a brief shift toward more organized health care structure and financing. However, the 1994 failure of the Clinton health care proposal, combined with consumer resistance, put the brakes on plans for large-scale reform (Oberlander, 2007). Since then, more coordinated systems of care have developed as a result of increased regulatory and reporting requirements, as well as changes in the reimbursement system toward consolidation driven by rising health care costs. Despite such financial consolidation, true clinical integration has materialized only among a minority of providers overall, within a largely fragmented health care landscape.

The increase in longevity related to medical progress, coinciding with the aging of the Baby Boomers, has led to a significant demographic shift in which a larger percentage of elderly patients live with more complex chronic disease. Since the early 1900s, the average lifespan has increased by more than 30 years (Penn Wharton Budget Model, 2016). These demographic changes have brought into stark relief the inherent cost and quality issues of our fragmented delivery system, intensifying the urgency of instituting dynamic and significant changes in that delivery system. The population of Americans aged 65 and older will reach more than 71 million by the time the last round of Baby Boomers reaches 65, according to a 2016 Census Bureau report on aging, signifying a 73% increase from the approximately 41 million in 2011 (Barr, 2014). The shift from commercial insurance to Medicare that many of these adults will make during that period threatens to place even greater strain on the Medicare system and federal budget. The anticipated effects of these trends in aging and longevity have driven a massive initiative to find new reimbursement models for Medicare along with all other insurance payers. This chapter will review some of the significant changes planned in multiple dimensions of our health care system.

II.   System dimensions and integration

Health care's transition from a fragmented cottage industry to an integrated clinical delivery system has left an impact in every corner of health care. The advent of this more complex landscape has given rise to horizontal and vertical integration of care. Horizontal integration links together providers at the same tier of the health care system to create economies of scale, such as partnerships between hospitals, consolidation of physicians with a single specialization into one practice, or creation of a national nursing home chain. Vertical integration links together providers whose roles lie at various levels of the health care system to provide a multitude of services under one umbrella, such as outpatient practitioners, hospitals, rehabilitation facilities, and even insurers and payers (Essential Hospitals Institute, 2013). Kaiser Permanente is a good example of an organization that is completely integrated on both horizontal and vertical planes.

Although the concept of horizontal and vertical integration is most often used in reference to business strategies, these terms also apply to strategies for clinical coordination of care, which requires inter-professional, interdisciplinary, and inter-sectoral collaboration across the diverse sites and disciplines engaged within a patient-care ecosystem. Such horizontal and vertical integration involves communication and coordination across multiple venues and care dimensions, which can be accomplished through both direct physical and virtual (electronic) connectivity. The development of hospital networks, single-specialty and multi-specialty practices, and independent practice associations have provided both geographic proximity and electronic coordination through common electronic medical records (EMRs), documentation systems for ancillary services, and electronic messaging capabilities, resulting in better communication channels for the coordination and integration of care.

The rise of specialty and hospital-based inpatient care shifted the paradigm for health care delivery as well. Such changes in models of care and delivery mechanisms did not translate into changes in defined roles and responsibilities when it came to ensuring accountability and communication. Instead, system-wide communication gaps, errors during transitions in care, and a generalized lack of accountability and responsibility became standard. This inefficient, costly and fragmented system provided a sub-optimal quality of care, marred by errors and preventable safety hazards, as recognized by the Institute of Medicine report, *To Err Is Human*, from November 1999 (Institute of Medicine, 1999). The Institute of Medicine report indicated that the U.S. health care system would require significant changes to achieve an adequate level of safety and quality, especially assigning clear responsibilities for communication and accountability and developing organized systems to improve performance. These systemic changes require planning processes of their own, if they are to be integrated and have maximum impact. Subsequent sections will highlight some of these developments.

A.   Preventive health and population management—Changing role of the health care system

Scientific advancements in medicine and the demographic changes as a result of the aging Baby Boomers have resulted in more patients living longer with chronic disease, which in turn has led to structural changes such as integration of care systems. But an even larger paradigm shift is required when it comes to the guiding philosophies for the medical profession, that would move physicians from an individual doctor-patient dynamic to a public health mind-set. Under the Hippocratic paradigm, a physician viewed patients on an individual level, with the goal of treating their particular medical concerns. This was based on a model of professional obligation and payment for services sought and rendered. A more modern, preventive, and population-based paradigm, in which government agencies and health researchers work toward a common goal of maintaining the general health of the overall population, has evolved from public health theory. As part of such a public health framework, researchers aggregate patients into demographic and epidemiological cohorts in order to better understand patterns of disease among specific populations, and policy experts recommend measures to improve the general health of the population such as sanitation, safe public water, and quarantines (Kluge, 2007). Placing individual physicians within a public health framework assigns responsibility to practitioners for the general health of their patient population, through systematic efforts applied on an individual basis. The obligations of providers, traditionally confined to curing illness, expand to encompass the promotion and maintenance of health through preventative health measures and screenings. Rather than treating illness only once it presents itself, physicians prevent its onset, identify it earlier, or slow the progression of chronic illness to avoid associated morbidities and complications. A provider thus no longer bears responsibility solely for individual patients, but for the health of a defined patient population, regardless of whether they seek care or currently have any illness. Patients can be contacted by outreach letter, email, or phone with reminders to obtain preventive screenings and recommended chronic disease management measures. These issues are addressed at every in-person contact regardless of the reason for the visit.

This modern approach promotes healthy behaviors and encourages behavioral changes that support wellness, including proactive interventions based on a patient's known risk factors. The success of a public health approach depends upon the rigorous collection and analysis of patient information, and segmentation of the population to define necessary interventions. The scientific-based paradigm in medicine has supported the transition to evidence-based medicine (EBM), defined as "a systematic approach to clinical problem solving that allows the integration of the best available research with clinical expertise and patient values" (Sackett, Trauss, & Richardson, 2000). EBM has been a powerful tool for population and preventative medicine. Before its rise in the twentieth century, the majority of medical practices had never been scientifically proven, instead based more on traditional "expert opinions" and informal experiences than randomized controlled studies or verification. More rigorous large population-based research, such as the longitudinal Framingham study, and controlled treatment studies, have established proven interventions that individual physicians could apply in their care for patients (Framingham Heart Study, 1948). Coupling these findings with advancements in information technology, including the large-scale deployment of electronic medical records, digitalization of health-care information, and application of sophisticated data analytics, today the health care system can deploy powerful tools to conduct research and manage health care. Such application of evidence-based preventive approaches, and a population-management approach making use of sophisticated data, empowers doctors and health care professionals to better manage individual- and population-level health.

While benefiting from evidence-based population knowledge and the added perspective of a global population-management framework (1:n), the physician faces the challenge of balancing these new norms with the historical Hippocratic-based (1:1) paradigm, a critical part of the professional trust required in the individual physician-patient relationship. Data gleaned from population medicine provide only statistical odds, not certainty, for any individual patient. The possibility always exists for individuals to have significant critical differences compared to the population pool, which would change their predictive risk. The acknowledgement and management of this variability can present an opportunity, rather than conflict, if physicians can synthesize a new dynamic role in constituting a new "art of medicine." This role of physician as problem framer requires a dialectic between the Hippocratic and population-based models. The physician first must use his/her professional expertise to identify important variations from the population norm, and then educate the patient on the predictive risk based on available evidence-based medical knowledge. Ultimately, having evaluated the patient's individual circumstances, the physician will engage in an educated, shared decision-making process that incorporates the patients' priorities, values, and goals of care.

B.   The health care team

Advances in medical knowledge and the growing complexity of therapeutics and interventions have resulted in another paradigm shift in the delivery of health care at the practitioner level: doctors now serve as leader within a team of integrated providers, rather than the focal source of a patient's medical care. Health care for the elderly, who require a multi-disciplinary approach to treating the more complex levels of disease that accompany the aging process, epitomizes this phenomenon. Traditionally, health care operated under a principle that viewed physicians as the sole deliverers, with other providers playing only minor supportive roles that lacked decision-making authority and autonomy outside of fulfilling a doctor's orders. The new, more complex health landscape, marked by an expansion of knowledge and the rise of evidence-based interventions, has transformed what had been a solo enterprise into a team sport. It is no longer feasible or logistically possible for an individual physician to provide the full spectrum of care for patients with multiple co-morbidities. As noted by Captain Chesley Burnett "Sully"

Sullenberger III, the pilot responsible for the "Miracle on the Hudson," the change in physicians' roles parallels the differences between pilots of a fighter jet versus a bomber (American Medical Group Association, 2013). While the physician still holds ultimate responsibility over a patient, the physician is now more akin to a team leader who provides direction and strategy. Other members of the team (nurse practitioner, physician's assistant, nurse, medical assistant, physical therapist, mental health therapist, nutritionist, health coach, etc.) play more important roles by providing monitoring, therapeutic interventions, teaching and recommendations, all critical to the patient's health outcomes and essential to the decision-making process (Bodenheimer & Bauer, 2016). The team approach will only rise in currency for its ability to address physician shortages, meet growing demand for health care, and dispense therapeutics and interventions with expanded capabilities. The shortage of physicians is particularly severe in primary care, especially in rural areas that face shortages of specialty physicians and other non-physician specialists (Markit, 2017). This shortage has also been exacerbated by the wave of retiring physicians in the Baby Boom generation and the profession's demographic shift toward a female majority of medical school graduates, who on average work fewer hours per week than their male predecessors (Markit, 2017). The current dictum in health care recommends a re-organization of clinical work to make the most effective use of one's medical license and training, so that everyone can function at the highest level possible.

The team concept goes further to include the patient as an active member, in contrast to their traditional status as a passive recipient of care. Given the widespread recognition of lifestyle and behavior as major factors in preventing and treating illness, as well as the knowledge that a patient's level of compliance can constitute a major barrier to successful therapeutic interventions, the patient's own actions become critical. The medical establishment has begun to challenge the patriarchal model in which patients passively accept physicians' decisions, with no involvement in the process. In its place, a more collaborative doctor-patient dynamic has emerged, bolstered by higher health literacy as a result of the Internet. Patients are more directly involved in their own medical decisions, combining physician's recommendations with their personal values and priorities. The physician's role has changed from a patriarchal problem-solver to a professional with expertise and experience, who can frame problems in context as part of a joint decision-making process. This emphasis on engaging patients in their treatment through shared decision making elevates them to the role of assuming responsibilities that serve as critical linchpins for their health. In circumstances where cognitive, cultural, or medical factors prevent patients from assuming a more active role, designated health care agents or caregivers enter the decision-making process as well. To be successful, physicians and the other members of the team will need to be trained in the skills necessary for effective education, behavioral interviewing, motivation, and engagement of their patients.

C. Medical home

The ascent of specialization over the last 50 years effectively marginalized the role of the primary care physician. The fee-for-service reimbursement model, developed under Medicare and commercial insurance programs in the 1960s, favored procedurally-oriented specialties through greater reimbursements, resulting in significantly higher prestige and incomes for specialists. A specialist can earn $3.5 million more than a primary care physician over the course of their career (Robert Graham Center, 2009). Since then, a larger percentage of medical school graduates have pursued specialties with fewer medical school graduates choosing primary care, culminating in a significant shortage of primary care physicians. Under every combination of scenarios modeled, the United States will face a worsening shortage of physicians over the next decade, according to a physician workforce report recently released by the Association of American Medical Colleges. The study estimates a shortfall of up to 43,000 primary care physicians by 2030 (Markit, 2017). As noted in the American Academy of Family Physicians' annual national study on the percentage of graduates pursuing various specialties, only 10% in 2016 selected family medicine (Kozakowski, Travis, Bentley, & Fetter, 2016). As outlined earlier, the fragmented system resulting from the shift toward specialization severed the primary care physician's connecting role as communicator and coordinator.

The concept of the medical home, which arose from the American Academy of Pediatrics during the 1970s and 1980s and involved the idea that the primary care physician would serve as "home base" for different types of care, came to prominence in response to the health care system's increasingly fractured dynamic. Subsequently, the American College of Family Physicians adopted the medical home model, followed by the American College of Physicians' internal medicine professional societies. Medicare and most commercial insurance companies have promoted the concept as a means to improve the quality and cost of care. Although its principles have evolved over time, the home model re-establishes the primary care physician (PCP) as the focal point for clinical information and oversight of the patient's total medical care. Embodying a holistic perspective that includes medical and psychosocial needs, it relies on the primary care physician to foster a long-term comprehensive relationship with the patient as the central coordinator for all medical needs. The PCP serves as an advocate to guide patients through the complex maze of the medical system and through the critical decision-making process during the course of illness (Robert Graham Center, 2007).

The medical home model epitomizes many of the principles and components of the modern delivery system outlined in other subsections of this chapter. The core of the "home" is the integration of information across the multiple venues and specialties that make up a patient's clinical course, providing continuity over that patient's lifetime. This long-term relationship supports the whole patient, including their social and family context and their psychosocial well being. The PCP, who serves as this medical home, also actively provides a preventive and population-based approach to patient care. Such a PCP acts as the leader of a multidisciplinary team that includes significant, active roles for mid-level providers, nurses, care managers, nutritionists, medical assistants, and health care coaches, among other disciplines that may be based in the medical home office. To increase the supply of PCPs, it will be necessary for PCP incomes to be more competitive with other specialties. This can be accomplished through changes in the reimbursement model that increase the reimbursement of cognitive non-procedural specialties and better reflect the value of their integrative role. This can be accomplished by compensating PCPs directly for the time they devote to the vital care coordination role, a role which was previously not reimbursable, though Medicare and commercial carriers are now beginning to offer reimbursement. In addition, the distribution of value-based reimbursement bonuses must be weighted to reflect the central role of the PCPs in these outcomes.

D.   Subacute and long-term care

With the increased longevity of the Baby Boomers, long-term care affects a large percentage of the aging population and represents a growing percentage of all health care costs. The number of elderly Americans who are 65 and older is projected to increase from 13% of the overall U.S. population in 2000, to 20% of the overall U.S. population in 2030 (Spillman, 2000). The implications for health care expenditures may be profound, given the significant increase in the use of nursing home services with longevity and the expense of institutional care:

> Total expenditures in 1996 dollars from the age of 65 years until death increase substantially with longevity from $31,181 for persons who die at the age of 65 years to more than $200,000 for those who die at the age of 90, in part because of steep increases in nursing home expenditures for very old persons.
>
> (Spillman, 2000)

The boom in the elderly population has put pressure on institutions and providers and prompted significant changes in this component of the delivery system. Traditional nursing homes have seen falling numbers of residents, the result of more people aging in place, along with reductions in reimbursement. New outpatient support structures and technology enable more patients to age in their homes until their medical needs require the support of a facility. The rise of AARP's "livable communities" initiative and services from other community-based and church-based nonprofit support organizations have further helped older people live in their homes rather than institutions. These groups provide social and logistical support and help with food and transportation, performing a function previously carried out most often by extended family.

Other models appeal to healthier, higher-functioning patients who still need more support or monitoring than they could receive at home, such as assisted living facilities and the newer Green House (GH) Project model (Robert Wood Johnson Foundation, 2017). These types of chronic care facilities provide patients greater autonomy in an environment that is more attractive than the traditional nursing home.

The GH model was developed by Dr. Bill Thomas, an innovative gerontologist, and the Robert Wood Johnson Foundation to provide a new model for long-term care that emphasizes autonomy and agency. The GH model observes a mission of providing its "elders," the program's term for residents, opportunities to build a meaningful life with a versatile, supportive staff and a real home setting. Green Houses are trademarked and built to strict standards. Adopters must agree to specific architectural requirements and workforce practices, including a flattened workforce hierarchy. The GH is committed to providing the structure and support to serve as a home for life, as long as each elder wishes to remain.

In this context of shrinking revenues and downsized patient populations, chronic care facilities and nursing homes that previously provided mostly low-level custodial support are developing the capacity to provide higher-level medical care, including nursing, intravenous fluid replacement, and provision of antibiotics and physical therapy. This shift has allowed them to compete for subacute care patients' post-hospitalization phase while managing their new primary demographic: higher-intensity chronic care patients.

E. Continuum of care

The fragmentation of the health care system has led to ineffective handoffs and communication during patient transitions across the continuum of care, from outpatient to hospital to subacute rehabilitation to nursing home, and finally to the community for outpatient care. Transitions have been identified as a major source of errors and gaps in care, resulting in failed treatment plans and patient decompensation, which then lead to complications and hospital readmissions. As the famous quote from the movie *Cool Hand Luke* goes, "What we've got here is failure to communicate." A major principle of the quality and safety movement is that structural handoffs, such as those occurring in transitions of care from one structural setting to another, are transactions with a high risk of failure. Thus, there are high stakes associated with these transitions, which demand special attention.

Until recently, only minimal efforts were made to solve these deficiencies, as neither party involved in patient transactions had the proper incentives to address the pitfalls of transitions. In fact, institutions profited from the readmissions. Through provisions in the Affordable Care Act, payers have focused attention on reducing readmissions by financially penalizing hospitals for poor management of transitions of care or failure to reduce readmissions. Quality management and safety techniques, developed to ensure that providers share information with one another, have been applied to transitions in order to eliminate some of the gaps in care. Electronic interfaces and electronic medical records (EMRs), and even hard copy or fax, have proved useful in addressing some of these perils of transition, although the lack of standardized interoperability or regional information networks hinders more widespread information sharing. Furthermore, both hospitals and ambulatory practitioners deploy additional resources in following up with patients and providers post-transition, to ensure that patients don't fall through the cracks. As the health care industry increasingly consolidates through vertical and horizontal integration, more seamless transitions can be organized and facilitated within a shared infrastructure.

F.   Quality and safety

The transformation of health care from an unsophisticated cottage industry to a sector with comprehensive organizational structures has brought to medicine the disciplines of quality and safety improvement. These modern approaches, which other industries had started assimilating into their guiding business principles in the mid-twentieth century, were foreign to health care. Disciplines such as "Total Quality Management" and "Continuous Quality Improvement" had significantly reduced errors, increased efficiency, and generated consistent outcomes in other fields such as manufacturing and the airline industry. The management theorist W. Edwards Deming introduced the technique of statistical process control to Japanese industries after World War II, a method that evolved into the Total Quality Management (TQM) approach, which focuses on efficient process, customer satisfaction, employee empowerment, and constant communication at all levels (Hashmi, 2017). U.S. industry and manufacturing began adopting these techniques in the 1980s, but only in the 1990s did the concept gain traction in health care organizations large enough for the methodology to be applicable and logistically feasible. Following the recommendations of Dr. Don Berwick and his organization, the Institute for Healthcare Improvement (IHI), most hospitals and larger health care provider groups have adopted some variation of quality practices that incorporate the principles of TQM, Continuous Quality Improvement (CQI), Six Sigma, the Toyota Way, or similar management philosophies. The Institute of Medicine's groundbreaking 1999 report, *To Err Is Human*, resulted in major safety initiatives in all health care institutions nationwide (Institute of Medicine, 1999).

Today, all governmental payers, insurance companies, hospital systems, and larger physician practices have formal quality and safety programs organized around the principles of quality management. These projects center on achieving targeted quality goals and reducing system errors.

G. *Palliative care and hospice*

Technological advancements have rendered many chronic diseases manageable for prolonged periods, changing the trajectory of a patient's illness. In earlier times, when medicine had a more limited armamentarium, patients with these same chronic illnesses typically followed an acute course of rapid deterioration and death. For the first time, older people with severe chronic diseases are experiencing prolonged periods of stable illness with associated symptomatology and suffering, elevating the importance of devoting more focus to well being, quality of life, and development as whole people rather than focusing care plans exclusively on treating and curing their illness medically.

Historically, the extended family provided most end-of-life care. Religious institutions served this role mainly for those with limited resources and no families. Soldiers in the Crusades set up the first homes for the incurably ill in the eleventh century, and the Knights Hospitaller, a religious order, opened a hospice-type facility in the fourteenth century to provide refuge for travelers and care for the terminally ill (Smith, 2012). Hospice is derived from the Latin *hospes*, which referred to either a travelling guest or host (Cass, 2015). Through the Middle Ages and the eighteenth and nineteenth centuries, religious orders administered most terminal care and hospice care outside of the family home, focusing predominantly on people with incurable illnesses.

The founder of the modern hospice movement, British physician Dame Cicely Saunders, first applied the term to specialized care for dying patients. She began her work with the terminally ill in 1948 and founded the first modern hospice, St. Christopher's Hospice in London, in 1967. A lecture she delivered at the Yale School of Nursing in 1965 introduced the United States to the concept. Less than a decade later in 1974, the first hospice in America, Connecticut Hospice, opened its doors, less than ten miles away from Yale in Branford, Connecticut (Connecticut Hospice, n.d.).

About hospice, the National Hospice and Palliative Care Organization says:

> It is considered to be the model for quality, compassionate care for people facing a life-limiting illness or injury, hospice care involves a team-oriented approach to expert medical care, pain management, and emotional and spiritual support expressly tailored to the patient's needs and wishes.
>
> (National Hospice and Palliative Care Organization, 2017)

The federal Health Care Financing Administration (HCFA) initiated a hospice demonstration program in 1979. Congress created a Medicare hospice benefit in 1982 that became permanent in 1986. States could opt to include hospice in their Medicaid programs, establishing a "hospice benefit" defined by certain criteria, including a prognosis of less than six months and cessation of curative treatments. By regulatory definition, then, hospice benefit became a narrow subset of what previously had been defined as palliative or hospice care. While hospice originated as a method of care for incurably ill people, its humanistic, holistic, team approach came to be defined more broadly under the umbrella of palliative care. Hospice care, not the "hospice benefit" of Medicare, refers to the subset of palliative care focused on end-of-life care for individuals with terminal illness. However, a person-centered holistic approach to medicine applies universally at all levels of patient care and should arguably be a norm for all interactions in the health care system, not only at the end of life. The specific significance and stage of the illness would then determine the balance between disease treatment and efforts towards symptom control and addressing the psychosocial impact of illness. The principles behind the palliative model share significant overlap with the aims of geriatric medicine, which addresses the broad spectrum of illness among older adults, from common aging disorders such as vision or hearing impairment, to multi-morbidity of chronic medical diagnoses, to frailty, vulnerability, and loss of function of activities of daily living. A growing movement proposes the integration of geriatrics and palliative care into a field known as *GeriPal*. From a broader perspective, palliative care embodies many principles of the modern clinical delivery system discussed in this chapter.

III. Conclusion

In response to the aging demographic of the largest generation in history, advancements in modern medicine, and economic pressures, the U.S. health system has evolved to develop new delivery system models and paradigms for health care. These care models focus on correcting deficiencies in the historically physician-centric, siloed, fragmented health care delivery system, which was inadequately equipped to address the increasing complexity and severity of illness among the aging population in this country. These models, created with the goal of improving the integration and coordination of care, are present to varying degrees in the following philosophies and principles:

- Person-centered care
- Coordinated team approach
- Proactive preventive care and population-based health management
- Medical protocols informed by evidence-based medicine
- Goals of care tailored to patients' needs and wishes
- Shared decision making
- Integration of continuum of care across the health care ecosystem

As our delivery system evolves to include new models or variations of older models, these themes will remain essential and critical dimensions of a modern health care delivery system capable of providing quality care.

References

American College of Healthcare Executives. (2007). History of health insurance in the United States. Retrieved December 1, 2017 from: www.ache.org>pubs>Morrisey 2253_Chapter1.pdf

American Medical Group Association (AMGA). (2013, March). *What the health care industry can learn from aviation.* Unpublished speech, 2013 Annual Conference.

Barr, P. (2014, January). Baby Boomers will transform health care as they age. *Hospital and Health Networks.* Retrieved August 25, 2017 from: www.hhnmag .com/articles/5298-Boomers-Will-Transform-Health-Care-as-They-Age

Bodenheimer, T., & Bauer, L. (2016). Rethinking the primary care workforce – An expanded role for nurses. *New England Journal of Medicine, 375*(11), 1015–1017. Retrieved October 21, 2017 from: www.nejm.org/doi/full/10.1056/NEJMp1606869

Cass, S. (2015). *A good death: A practical guide to maintaining control of your end-of-life journey.* Bloomington, IN: Balboa Press.

Committee on the Governance and Financing of Graduate Medical Education. (2014). Graduate medical education that meets the nation's health needs. Retrieved July 31, 2017 from: www.ncbi.nlm.nih.gov/books/NBK248023/

Connecticut Hospice Inc. (n.d). History of the Connecticut Hospice. Retrieved May 2017 from: www.hospice.com/about/timeline/

Essential Hospitals Institute. (2013). Integrated healthcare literature review. Retrieved December 4, 2017 from: www.essentialhospitals.org/wp-content/uploads/2013/12 /Integrated-Health-Care-Literature-Review-Webpost-8-22-13-CB.pdf

Framingham Heart Study. (1948). Retrieved August 13, 2017 from: www.framingham heartstudy.org

Hashmi, K. (2017). Introduction and implementation of total quality management (TQM). Retrieved July 15, 2017 from: www.isixsigma.com/methodology/total -quality-management-tqm/introduction-and-implementation-total-quality-man agement-tqm/

Institute of Medicine (IOM). (1999). *To err is human: Building a safer health system.* Retrieved July 15, 2017 from: www.ncbi.nlm.nih.gov/pubmed/25077248

Institute of Medicine (IOM). (2008). *Retooling for an aging America: Building the health care workforce.* Washington, DC: The National Academic Press.

Kluge, E.W. (2007). Resource allocation in healthcare: Implications of models of medicine as a profession. *Medscape General Medicine, 9*(1), 57. Retrieved December 6, 2017 from: www.medscape.com/viewarticle/551802_5

Kozakowski, S. Travis, A., Bentley, A., & Fetter, G. (2016). Entry of US medical school graduates into family medicine residencies: 2015–2016. *Family Medicine, 48*(9), 688–695. Retrieved July 15, 2017 from: www.stfm.org/FamilyMedicine/Vol48 Issue9/Kozakowski688

Markit, I.H.S. (2017, February 28). *Update: The complexities of physician supply and demand: Projections from 2015 to 2030.* Report prepared for the Association of American Medical Colleges. Retrieved December 6, 2017 from: https://aamc-black .global.ssl.fastly.net/production/media/filer_public/a5/c3/a5c3d565-14ec-48fb -974b-99fafaeecb00/aamc_projections_update_2017.pdf

National Hospice and Palliative Care Organization. (2017, April 3). Hospice care. Retrieved May 2017 from: www.nhpco.org/about/hospice-care

Oberlander, J. (2007). Learning from failure in health care reform. *New England Journal of Medicine, 357,* 1677–1679. Retrieved November 28, 2017 from: www .nejm.org/doi/full/10.1056/NEJMp078201

Penn Wharton Budget Model. (2016, June 27). Mortality in the United States: Past, present and future. Retrieved December 5, 2017 from: http://budgetmodel.wharton .upenn.edu/issues/2016/1/25/mortality-in-the-united-states-past-present-and-future

Ringel, J.S., Hosek, S.D., Vollaard, B.A., & Mahnovskiet, S. (2002). The elasticity of demand for health care: A review of the literature and its application to the military health system. Retrieved December 5, 2017 from: www.rand.org/pubs/mono graph_reports/MR1355.html

Robert Graham Center. (2007, November). The patient-centered medical home: History, seven core features, evidence and transformational change. Retrieved December 5, 2017 from: www.aafp.org>dam>initiatives>PCMH.pdf

Robert Graham Center. (2009). What influences medical student and resident choices? Retrieved December 3, 2017 from: www.graham-center.org/content/dam/rgc/docu ments/publications-reports/monographs-books/Specialty-geography-compressed .pdf

Robert Wood Johnson Foundation. (2017). The Green House Project: Reimagining traditional nursing homes. Retrieved July 15, 2017 from: www.rwjf.org/en/how-we -work/grants-explorer/featured-programs/the-green-house-project.html

Rosenberg, C.E. (1987). *The care of strangers: The rise of hospital systems.* New York: Basic Books. Retrieved December 1, 2017 from: www.ncbi.nlm.nih.gov /pmcarticles/PMC4

Sackett, D.L, Trauss, S.E., & Richardson, W.S. (2000). *Evidence-based medicine: How to practice and teach EBM, (2nd ed).* Edinburgh: Churchill Livingstone.

Smith, C.E. (2012). *A hospice guide book.* Bloomington, IN: Inspiring Voices.

Spillman, B.C., & Lubitz, J. (2000). The effect of longevity on spending for acute and long-term care. *New England Journal of Medicine, 342*(19), 1409–1415. Retrieved December 5, 2017 from: www.nejm.org/doi/full/10.1056/NEJ M20000511342906

5 Evolution of financing models and impact on quality and services for older adults

I. Introduction: Financing, reimbursement, and cost-saving models

The financing of health care has implications for the functioning of the health care system at all levels. From the source of insurance coverage and the purview of people and services that are covered, to the reimbursement model that determines how services are purchased and valued, these variables have an immense impact on the scope and quality of the health care received in the United States. Each of these areas has evolved over the last six decades and continues to evolve as our society responds to changes in the economic environment and a desire to fine tune and improve the current system.

II. Insurance financing and coverage

The source and degree of funding for insurance determines who has coverage, which in turn determines the scope of medical care available to an individual. Prior to the late 1940s and 1950s, approximately 80% of individuals had no health insurance coverage and paid for services privately (Conover, 2011). The expansion of medical knowledge, diagnostics, and therapeutics in the 1950s and 1960s necessitated more hospital-based care (Rosenberg, 1987). A significant rise in the cost of care for serious illness, beyond the financial wherewithal of most individuals, accompanied these advances in medical sophistication. Federal wage controls during World War II led employers to offer private health insurance as a benefit to circumvent the cap on employee pay, ushering in the widespread use of employer-paid health insurance. Employers continued to offer insurance policies as a recruitment tool after the wage limits expired, and labor unions pushed for companies to provide health insurance policies for workers. Commercial insurance was then also available on a private basis to individuals who could afford the cost if their employers did not cover them (Rank, 2017). This patchwork created different levels of coverage, including individuals who lacked any coverage. Included in the uninsured were a large percentage of elder Americans who were no longer employed, as well as low-income or unemployed individuals.

The signing of the original Medicare and Medicaid Act on July 30, 1965 by President Lyndon Johnson addressed the disproportionate lack of insurance among older and low-income individuals (Berkowitz, 2008). The legislation guaranteed health insurance for Americans aged 65 and older, which ultimately reduced the number of uninsured to below 20% in the 1970s (Conover, 2011). It was predominantly financed by a Medicare-specific payroll tax on working individuals and their employers. In addition, the Act created Medicaid, a medical insurance program for citizens who met the legally defined criteria for poverty (U.S. Department of Health & Human Services, 2005). Medicaid was financed separately through a combination of state and federal funding, with states individually in control of their own benefit programs. This model has resulted in wide variations in the types of services and amount of funding available, leading for the most part to an inadequately funded, lower-tier health insurance program that largely provides less reimbursement and access to providers and services compared to private insurance policies. The single-payer, governmental structure of these programs effectively established health care as a de facto right for older and lower-income Americans, with the potential to be eventually expanded to all citizens. In subsequent years, these governmental programs incrementally expanded coverage to more categories of citizens under the Medicare and Medicaid umbrellas. The Medicare Prescription Drug Improvement and Modernization Act of 2003 broadened the Medicare program with the establishment of Part C and Part D. Part C created a financing structure for the government to fund and transfer insurance risk to approved private health plans, known as Medicare Advantage plans, thereby diverging from the single-payer model. Part D, structured to be administered and sold by private insurance plans rather than the government, expanded the scope of coverage to include medication costs (U.S. Department of Health & Human Services, 2005).

While most developed countries in the West have adopted the social ethic of basic health care as a fundamental right and provide various forms of universal health care coverage for their citizenry, following the 1965 passage of Medicaid and Medicare, the U.S. government did not approach that question until the Clinton administration put forth a plan for universal health care coverage in 1993. That proposal, the Health Security Act, ultimately foundered under significant lobbying resistance from the established health care industry, including hospitals, insurers, pharmaceutical companies, and physicians, as well as concerns among the American public regarding bureaucracy, competition in the marketplace, and individual freedom of choice (Oberlander, 2007). The 1997 passage of the Children's Health Insurance Program (CHIP), a limited vestige of the original Clinton health plan, expanded coverage as a right to uninsured children. In conjunction with Medicaid, CHIP covers one in three children in the United States and has cut the number of uninsured children in half since its enactment (Paradise, 2014). Nevertheless, this approach did not proceed further in the United States due to the aforementioned strength of opposing lobbying interests from the health care industry and the persistent American cultural biases against government programs and mandates.

The Affordable Care Act (ACA), while limited, moved America closer in the direction of universal coverage with its passage in 2010, making insurance more available for a wider segment of Americans and giving a platform to the concept of health care as a right rather than privilege. Under the ACA, the government established the structure, set regulations, and funded or subsidized portions of insurance premiums; however, the program predominantly acted through the private insurance market and delivery system rather than establishing a new government-funded insurance program. The ACA enabled a significant percentage of the previously uninsured to obtain health insurance through expanded subsidies, made children up to the age of 26 eligible to receive coverage through their parents' policies, removed pre-existing illness as a barrier to coverage, guaranteed transportability of coverage between places of employment, and introduced the exploration of new reimbursement models to control costs and improve quality, which will be examined in later sections of this book (Affordable Care Act, 2010).

Even with the development and expansion of these government-based insurance initiatives, the majority of insurance coverage in the United States—67.2% in 2015—is still provided by private commercial insurance companies (Barnett & Vornovitsky, 2016). To a certain extent, commercial carriers also participate in these government programs and share the risk for selected Medicare patients, specifically those with Medicare Advantage and Medicaid patients under capitation arrangements. The total number of uninsured Americans remained at 11.3% in the first quarter of 2017, down from 18% in 2008 (Auter, 2017). The United States still does not guarantee global health care coverage to its citizenry as a basic right. Despite the successes of the ACA, a significant political movement has risen up to repeal the legislation. The depth and complexity of its current implementation, as well as the popularity of many of its provisions, make the possibility of a total repeal politically and operationally difficult, but the threat of significant modifications, if not total repeal, will loom large in future years.

As currently structured, all insurance programs have varying degrees of coverage providing different levels of benefits. The original health care indemnity insurance and early HMO models, like Kaiser Permanente's earlier incarnations, paid for all authorized, medically necessary, covered expenses without deductibles or copays. Early indemnity and HMO insurance plans without copays and deductibles no longer exist due to the competitive nature of rising health care expenses and premiums. The levels of copays and deductibles now vary by the specifics of what is covered, who can provide the services, and how much of the costs patients are responsible for through deductibles and co-insurance. Most states have a minimum standard of what must be covered by licensed state insurance companies or plans qualified under ERISA, the Employee Retirement Income Security Act of 1974, which set minimum standards for private pension and insurance plans—although the copays and deductibles could vary (U.S. Department of Labor, 2017). The ACA set standard minimum-benefit levels and standardized the ranges of copays and deductibles for the different levels of plans to allow consumers to compare associated premiums. Rises in health care costs have led to a trend among employers to shift more of the expense onto their employees, increasing individuals' deductibles and copays and the employees' percentage of the premium (Kaiser Family Foundation, 2016). Other trends in the benefits arena include linking lower premiums to a narrower network of providers, and either reducing or eliminating coverage of non-emergent, out-of-network expenses. These trends have eliminated the historically inelastic economic model and price insensitivity of health care, whereby the consumers did not feel the financial impact of the direct cost of care. Previously, most costs had largely been paid by the insurers, whether private or government, and financed through the insurance premiums paid by employers or federal and state taxes. With consumers paying more directly out of pocket for premiums, and more first-dollar care—for example, deductibles increased from $735 on average in 2008 to an average of $1478 in 2016—the cost of health care has become more visible to the consumer (Kaiser Family Foundation, 2016). This growing direct financial impact is beginning to have an effect on consumer behavior and on decisions regarding insurance, choices of providers, and real-time medical decisions, as networks narrow and high-deductible health plans proliferate (Kaiser Family Foundation, 2016). This new cost consciousness resets the complex value equation for health care, which we will discuss later in the book (Kaiser Family Foundation, 2016).

III.   Reimbursement models

A.   *Hospital reimbursement model*

As outlined above, the shift towards more expensive, hospital-based medical care was the primary driver of the newfound need for health care insurance. Initially, health insurance companies functioned purely as a vehicle for paying claims. Hospitals independently set their charges, and insurance companies paid the bills for covered services. With the implementation of Medicare, a large governmental payor began to establish policies and principles underlying the reimbursement model. Initially, reimbursement was based on individual hospital cost reports and historical charges, with Medicare reimbursement levels pegged to reported expenses plus an additional factor for capital reinvestment and a margin for financial viability. This reimbursement model had no incentive for controlling costs, essentially "rewarding" some hospitals for inefficiency or heavy investments in capital expansion regardless of the documented need. Expenses were converted into an average cost per day, called a "per diem," which provided a further incentive for extended, inefficient, or unjustified hospital stays. These factors led toward a progressive increase in hospital expenses.

With the Tax Equity and Fiscal Responsibility Act (TEFRA) of 1982, a prospective payment system based on Diagnosis-Related Groupings (DRGs) was gradually introduced over three years and fully implemented in 1986 (Centers for Medicare & Medicaid Services, 2016). Under this new system, each individual hospital was reimbursed flat rates for each DRG, and these rates were weighted by various associated hospital characteristics such as historical geographic costs, teaching and research programs, and amount of uninsured health care provided. As commercial insurers began to manage their insurance costs more aggressively and negotiate with hospitals for contractually agreed rates, they generally used the Medicare pricing models as a basis for their negotiations. Relying on their market share and leverage, the insurance companies negotiated significantly lower contract rates with hospital facilities compared to the hospitals' full rates. Because the insurers had less market control and clout with the hospitals than Medicare, which unilaterally establishes its rate formula without negotiation, they also paid higher rates, with the result that the commercial market indirectly subsidized Medicare and Medicaid. With the consolidation of health insurers beginning in the early 2000s and accelerating over the last several years, individual commercial insurers in certain states have attained dominant market positions, allowing them to negotiate hospital reimbursement contracts for less than the government payors, thus reversing the direction of subsidization in many cases (America's Health Insurance Plans, 2016).

In addition to DRG payments, Medicare has also introduced quality- and value-based incentives to hospitals as part of its shift in emphasis toward value-based measurement and reimbursement models. These quality measures are now reported and compared transparently on the Medicare website, and performance on certain measures can affect individual hospital reimbursement (Centers for Medicare & Medicaid Services, 2017). Medicare has incorporated metrics for quality that include standards for processes of care, such as time elapsed from emergency room entry to initiation of antibiotic therapy for illnesses like pneumonia, or time to cardiac intervention from emergency room registration for heart attacks (Chassin, Loeb, Schmaltz, & Wachter, 2010). Medicare also defined "never events," a colloquialism for serious reportable events stemming from the fact that they should never happen, as particularly shocking medical errors that are adverse, unambiguous, serious, and usually preventable events such as wrong-side surgery, retained objects, and medication errors in prescribing or administering medication (Agency for Healthcare Research and Quality Patient Safety Network, 2017). In these cases, Medicare will deny reimbursement for associated medical costs. Medicare also monitors hospital readmissions and will not reimburse the cost of readmissions within 30 days regardless of the diagnosis, and if a hospital sees readmission rates above a certain level, it will reduce the level of its payments for that hospital. As part of the ACA mandate to explore alternative quality and reimbursement models, Medicare has piloted bundled payment models, in which treatment for specific diagnoses or defined episodes of care is reimbursed not as many separate services, but under a single umbrella. This approach has expanded the DRG model, which typically applies only to acute care, by including care outside of the hospital setting for extended periods of time. This payment model dramatically alters the hospital's orientation regarding discharge, the need for transitions of care, and communication with the delivery system outside the hospital. A system of payment that tracks the continuum of care could serve as a potential motivator for better hand-offs and partnerships between the inpatient institution and the ambulatory and outpatient delivery systems.

B.   Provider reimbursement models

The traditional U.S. model for provider reimbursement, fee-for-service, is a transaction-based system that ties reimbursement to the type and number of services provided. As mentioned in Chapter 4 on delivery systems, this model derives from the historical Hippocratic paradigm of contractual, one-to-one relationships with individual patients based on professional obligation and payment for services sought and rendered. The development of health insurance was not initially disruptive to this arrangement; instead, it was structured as an additional layer. As a simple insurance product that paid providers in exchange for a fixed premium, it spread the cost of health care among a pool of individuals, protecting against the risk of large costs associated with serious illness. Commercial health insurance became more prevalent, prompting insurers to compete on price and gain market clout and leverage. Insurers seeking more profitability began to insert themselves more aggressively into financial relationships with providers. Rather than simply reimbursing claims, they began contracting directly with these providers and negotiating discounted reimbursement rates, instead of reimbursing them at their standard fee schedule. These practices gradually developed in the late 1980s and early 1990s, beginning with primary care physicians and hospitals. Over time, as the insurers' leverage increased, the majority of physicians in each specialty began to participate with the major insurers under contracted rates (American College of Healthcare Executives, 2007). A small percentage (approximately 8%) of high-profile physicians with established reputations, particularly at academic centers, still do not accept insurance rates, choosing instead to receive payment from patients based on their own independently established fee schedules (Physicians Foundation, 2016). In addition, since the 2000s, a small number of primary care physicians have created concierge practices, which are structured to provide a higher level of service to a smaller number of patients. Here, the financial structure requires patients to pay an annual stipend that will either cover all medical services in the practice or serve as a complement to individual transactions for services. As physicians consolidated into larger financial entities during the 2000s, either as academic or group practices or as Independent Practice Associations (IPAs), the leverage has shifted back towards the provider side to varying degrees, depending on the size of the affiliated groups. Larger entities no longer accept providers' standard fee schedules, opting instead to negotiate special reimbursement rates that are in some cases significantly higher than the standard fees.

An alternative form of provider reimbursement that originated with the HMO insurance model was capitation. This model serves a defined population within a restricted network of providers who can provide services, a feature intrinsic to the HMO structure. In contrast to the transaction model, capitation provides a fixed payment to providers from the insurer for all services covering and administered to that defined group of people or population. Capitation can take the form of a partial model for a specific specialty like primary care or cardiology, or a global model that includes the majority of medical costs, depending on the scope of the contracting organization. Simple capitation models transfer the full risk of excess utilization to providers in the case of single-specialty capitation, or excess expenses in the case of global capitation. More sophisticated models could be structured to limit exposure to risk, with the inclusion of financial provisions for risk corridors or stop-loss insurance, which protect contracting entities from financial devastation if claims exceed capacity. These models are calculated on a per-member, per-month basis based on historic costs and projections for services, which are predetermined by the provider and the insurer (James & Poulson, 2016). Such technical provisions provided a buffer against excessive losses but were usually symmetrical when it came to both upside or downside variances, which also limited potential profit. As mentioned earlier, the HMO model seemed to be gaining traction for a period in the early 1990s. At the time, many thought that the capitation model was the wave of the future. However, the HMO model lost steam, both from the failure of Clinton-era health reform legislation in Congress and as a result of patient resistance to limited choice. Providers also became wary of capitation, after initial forays resulted in financial losses for provider groups who lacked the necessary sophistication in contracting, clinical care, and utilization management skills to be successful. The exception was California, where there was a longer history of larger group practices, independent physician associations, and exposure to the capitation model. Organizations there had already had an opportunity to develop their organizational structure and infrastructure in the 1970s, making capitation viable with successful medical groups such as Palo Alto Medical Clinic or HealthCare Partners Medical Group (Robinson & Casalino, 1995). California and other West Coast states were the only sections of the country where capitation continued to a significant degree after the 1990s.

Outside of the West Coast, fee-for-service reimbursement, predominantly through preferred provider organizations insurance structures—known as PPOs—became the dominant commercial insurance and reimbursement model through the late 1990s and first decade of the 2000s. This model included financial incentives for staying within the preferred network, but still provided coverage for non-preferred providers, albeit at a higher expense to the patient. Through this structure, insurers attempted to steer patients toward lower-cost contracted physicians and a lower unit cost of care but did not address the fundamental transaction model of fee-for-service which rewarded volume, not medical value.

Starting in 2013, the ACA pioneered a new reimbursement model for Medicare called Accountable Care Organizations (ACOs), which many commercial insurers began to pilot. Health care policy makers and insurers also began exploring the concept of pay-for-performance in the late 1990s and early 2000s. The insurers initially targeted the quality measures for their HMO patients, which rated and compared them with other insurers through the Healthcare Effectiveness Data and Information Set, known as HEDIS. These insurers offered physicians relatively modest bonus incentives designed to motivate them to improve their HEDIS outcomes, for which the former were competing. In 2006, at a Medicare Payment Advisory Committee (MEDPAC) meeting held to address concerns over both the rising health care costs for Medicare beneficiaries and an absence of focus on quality, Dr. Elliott Fisher—a distinguished academic and researcher regarding the health care system—first used the term Accountable Care Organization. He expounded on this further in a subsequent *Health Affairs* article in January 2007, defining an ACO as an entity that will be "held accountable" for providing comprehensive health services to a defined population (Fisher et al., 2007). This loosely defined group of providers would, in other words, be held to account for measured improvements in the cost and quality of health care delivered to a population. This goal of improving quality and lowering cost for a defined population is the essence of successful population health management. The ACA in 2010 further solidified the role of ACOs, authorizing the Centers for Medicare and Medicaid Services to create such a program by January of 2012. Although broadly defined under the ACA, the ACO was intended as an experimental pilot vehicle that would change the existing reimbursement model, aimed at improving quality while reducing costs. Its underlying premise of "pay-for-performance" encouraged a significant paradigm shift from a transaction-based, fee-for-service model to a value-based one. Value-based reimbursement models condition reimbursement levels on performance measures or outcomes that reflect the "value" or improvement in health outcomes, relative to cost produced by the services. In parallel, private insurers began experimenting with variations on this theme of adhering to value-focused principles, which they also referred to as ACOs. While these individual models sometimes differed in measures, benchmarks, target outcomes, and financial specifics, they all shared a similar intrinsic shift toward basing reimbursement on performance or value produced, rather than the volume of services. After several years of implementing the ACO model, Medicare is making changes to its financial rules and calculations in an effort to refine the system so that it is more fair and predictable. Private insurers' ACO models are also evolving based on their experience. While these structures may continue to evolve and even change nomenclature, there is a general consensus among legislative and health care experts that a transition from fee-for-service to some form of value-based reimbursement will be necessary over time in order to control the excessive cost of health care in the United States. As a percentage of GDP, U.S. health care spending is approximately double that in other developed countries, where there are also better population health outcomes (Commonwealth Fund Report, 2014). The resulting impacts on the competitive position of the U.S. economy and the federal budget will constitute an economic driving force for fundamental change in these policies, independent of the success of current ACO structures or the potential repeal of the ACA.

C.   Long-term care reimbursement models

The demographic expansion of the Baby Boomers and increase in longevity related to medical progress have vastly increased the number of patients living with chronic debilitating diseases. This in turn has led to a significant increase in demand for long-term services, with as much as a 75% increase in spending for these services, which are defined as "a continuum of medical and social services designed to support the needs of people living with chronic health problems that affect their ability to perform everyday activities," and include "traditional medical services, social services and housing" (Ng, Harrington, & Kitchener, 2010). Medicare coverage for long-term care is limited and restrictive, as it was not set up to provide extended long-term care unrelated to a specific acute cause (Eiken, Sredl, Burwell, & Gold, 2010). Medicare will cover long-term care only for specifically designated skilled services over and above personal care. For long-term care services in a skilled nursing facility, Medicare will cover up to 100 days—but only following a hospital stay of at least three days, and only if the patient requires daily skilled medical services such as wound care or physical therapy. For individuals certified as homebound, Medicare will provide intermittent skilled services such as skilled nursing, physical therapy, or speech therapy, and Medicare-approved durable medical equipment, with a 20% copay as of 2017. It will also cover long-term care under the hospice benefit, which offers a broader range of covered home services for patients deemed hospice-eligible, that is, with less than six months to live.

Meanwhile, for those who qualify with incomes and assets below the program's designated thresholds, Medicaid covers long-term care services in nursing homes and home-based, long-term care services, such as visiting nurses and assistance with personal care. Medicaid is the largest payer for long-term care in the United States, even though only 7% of recipients receive long-term care services (U.S. Department of Health & Human Services, 2017). Unlike Medicare, it pays for custodial services in nursing homes and at home, which accounts for about one-third of total Medicaid spending (Michael & Chernew, 2003). Under Medicaid's structure of joint federal and state funding, the federal government sets minimum eligibility requirements and benefits, and individual states can choose whether to expand eligibility and benefits beyond the federal baseline. Elderly patients who require long-term custodial care but do not qualify for Medicaid face financial strain, as do their families. These patients and their families have felt compelled in some cases to manipulate income and assets to qualify for Medicaid, so that they can receive such custodial care. Aside from paying for services out-of-pocket, private long-term care insurance policies remain an option. As Americans witness the financial stresses imposed by long-term care costs, or learn that Medicare does not cover such care, more individuals have begun to purchase long-term care insurance as protection against the significant expenses that could arise in their later years. However, these policies are relatively expensive, and offered by relatively few companies. The low profitability of the insurance led some companies to stop selling policies, whether from the choice to focus on more commercially viable types of insurance or because the company ceased operations altogether. As a result of this dwindling market, consumers currently have limited options for private long-term care insurance coverage (Gleckman, 2012).

IV.   Cost-saving models

Between 1945 and 1998, the growth rate in real per capita national health care spending averaged 4.1%, as compared with a 1.5% increase in GDP (Kaiser Family Foundation, 2016). Health care still represents an outsized part of the American economy: 17.8% of GDP in 2015, expected to increase to 20.1% by 2025. The U.S. health care system saw total spending of $3.2 trillion in 2015, or almost $10,000 for each person, according to the latest federal projections. Currently, health care costs rise at about 5.5% per year (Herman, 2016; see also Figure 5.1).

Ultimately, the ideal reimbursement model, regardless of its name or specific rules, should have a structure that incentivizes improvements in the quality and efficiency of the health care that patients receive. The transaction-based, fee-for-service system generally imposed no barriers for physicians when it came to performance or ordering services that they considered necessary for providing their patients the best care. On the other hand, this carried the potentially perverse incentive of rewarding the number of services, regardless of their necessity or value to the patient (Miller, 2007). More care is not always better care. Every intervention has a potential for side effects, patient anxiety and false positives, or ambivalent results, which can then lead to further unnecessary interventions with their own risks for negative sequelae. In addition, under the fee-for-service model there was no intrinsic incentive for physicians to consider the added value versus cost of care, except where the patient's insurance did not sufficiently cover the charges. In contrast, classic capitation gives physicians an incentive to control utilization and costs, but also comes with potential perverse incentives to withhold appropriate care as a cost-saving measure. Additionally, this model has no built-in protections to ensure quality of care. Traditional efforts on the part of insurance companies

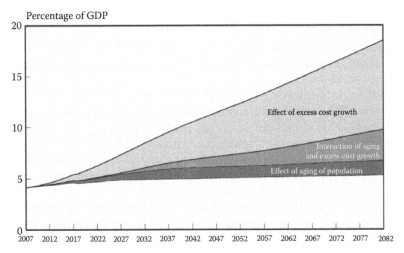

Percentage of GDP

Effect of excess cost growth

Interaction of aging and excess cost growth

Effect of aging of population

- It is the rate of spending per individual that will have the most impact, rather than the quantity / demographics of an aging population.
- "Excess cost growth" refers to the extent to which the increase in health care spending for an average individual exceeds the growth in per capita GDP.
- "Interaction…" refers to effects of excess cost growth and the aging of the population, which result in greater growth in spending than would result from either factor separately.
- "Aging of population" refers to demographic shifts, such as an increasing average population age and life expectancy.

Figure 5.1 Projected federal spending on Medicare and Medicaid (% GDP). *Source*: Congressional Budget Office.

to control costs through lowering of reimbursement levels, thereby reducing unit cost—or requiring preapproval, thereby reducing the volume of services—had only very limited and short-term effects.

However, the scale of cost reduction needed to make delivery of high-quality universal health care financially sustainable on an economic and societal level requires transformations that go beyond reimbursement models. The American health care system needs to see fundamental alterations in the processes of care delivery itself. Front-loaded investments in preventive care akin to the ACA's elimination of copays for preventive care, and incentives to promote healthier lifestyles or behavioral changes, can reap large benefits in long-term savings. Such a holistic shift will require a global, long-term perspective as opposed to the current short-term, siloed approach. An integrated systems approach, similar in concept to Total Quality Management in business, would provide a larger sphere of control and greater accountability. Otherwise, cost savings within one silo may simply lead to extra costs within other silos. Not providing home care visits for frail home-bound patients with more complex conditions will eventually result in hospital costs that exceed the home care costs. By the same token, under more siloed organizational and financial models, the investment in a small extra cost within a single silo cannot reap the reward of larger system-wide gains in quality and cost reduction. Additional outpatient expenses on home visits will not be counterbalanced by savings in inpatient hospital costs, if those savings are not distributed throughout the expanded universe of care.

In addition, new paradigms of care delivery that leverage new technology and seek to modernize near-sacrosanct historical practices of medicine, such as cardiac treatment, need to be piloted and tested. The history of medicine since the 1980s has shown dramatic improvements in quality and efficiency. Researchers have challenged historical practices that lacked evidence-based foundations and piloted new approaches that have proven themselves superior. Moreover, studies have demonstrated that many of those older approaches were not merely less effective and efficient, but actively harmful, whereas innovative approaches once considered experimental showed documented improvements in outcomes. Treatment of acute myocardial infarctions illustrates a classic example of this narrative. During the 1960s and 1970s, heart attack patients were typically treated with a month of bed rest; today, patients are mobilized out of bed in the first 24 to 48 hours. This change in practice has reduced incidence of venous thromboembolism and pulmonary emboli, pneumonia, cardiac and muscular deconditioning, bedsores, and other side-effects of prolonged bed rest with no deleterious effects and improved outcomes (Sharifi & Zeydi, 2016).

V.   Conclusion

The greatest promise for dramatic improvement lies in areas relating to system and process, where proven techniques of industrial-process improvement, adapted to take into account the special nature of relationships in the health care field, can be applied. These strategies improve efficiency and quality of hand-offs and transitions of care by applying the formal techniques of Total Quality Management to health care events that have historically been poorly managed and uncoordinated. Changes that further structural integration and alignment of incentives for all components of the system will advance the goal of improved quality and cost efficiency for patients in the United States. There is also untapped potential in a broader incorporation of the principles underlying different paradigms of care, such as the patient-centered medical home and the field of palliative medicine, both of which in some respects bring us back to the roots of medicine through their more holistic focus. Such a perspective transcends a technical focus on treating illnesses to embrace a more person-centered, humanistic understanding of patients, aimed at treating the whole person.

References

Affordable Care Act of 2010. (2010). Compilation of Patient Protection and Affordable Care Act. Publication No. 111–148, §2. Retrieved August 7, 2017 from: www.hhs .gov/sites/default/files/ppacacon.pdf

Agency for Healthcare Research and Quality Patient Safety Network. (2017). Never events. Retrieved December 1, 2017 from: https://psnet.ahrq.gov>primers>primer

American College of Healthcare Executives. (2007). History of health insurance in the United States. Retrieved December 1, 2017 from: www.ache .org>pubs>Morrisey2253_Chapter1.pdf

America's Health Insurance Plans (AHIP). (2016, February 17). National comparisons of commercial and Medicare fee-for-service payments to hospitals. Retrieved August 7, 2017 from: www.ahip.org/national-comparisons-of-commercial-and -medicare-fee-for-service-payments-to-hospitals/

Auter, Z. (2017, April 10). U.S. uninsured rate edges up slightly. Retrieved July 28, 2017 from: www.gallup.com/poll/208196/uninsured-rate-edges-slightly.aspx

Barnett, J.C., & Vornovitsky, M. (2016, September 13). Health insurance coverage in the United States: 2015. Retrieved July 2017 from: www.census.gov/library/publi cations/2016/demo/p60-257.html

Berkowitz, E. (2008). Medicare and Medicaid: The past as prologue. *Health Care Financing Review*, *29*(3), 81–93.

Casalino, L., & Robinson, J. (1997, September). The evolution of medical groups and capitation in California. Retrieved August 7, 2017 from: www.chcf.org/~/media /MEDIA%20LIBRARY%20Files/PDF/PDF%20C/PDF%20casalino.pdf

Centers for Medicare & Medicaid Services. (2016). Design and development of the Diagnosis Related Group (DRG) PBL-038. Retrieved December 1, 2017 from: www.cms.gov>fullcode_cms>Design_and_Development_of_the_Diagnosis _Related_Group_(DRG)

Centers for Medicare & Medicaid Services. (2017). Outcome measures. Retrieved December 1, 2017 from: www.cms.gov/Medicare/Quality-Initiatives-Patient -Assessment-Instruments/HospitalQualityInits/OutcomeMeasures.html

Centers for Medicare & Medicaid Services. (2017, January 1). *Outcome and assessment informations set: OASIS-C2 guidance manual*. Retrieved July 28, 2017 from: www.cms.gov/Medicare/Quality-Initiatives-Patient-Assessment-Instruments /HomeHealthQualityInits/Downloads/OASIS-C2-Guidance-Manual-6-17-16.pdf

Chassin, M.R., Loeb, J.M., Schmaltz, S.P., & Wachter, R.M. (2010). Accountability measures – Using measurements to promote quality improvement. *New England Journal of Medicine*, *363*, 683–688. Retrieved December 1, 2017 from: www.nejm .org/doi/full/10.1056/NEJMsb1002320#t=article

Commonwealth Fund. (2014). Healthcare spending as a percentage of GDP. Retrieved December 1, 2017 from: www.commonwealthfund.org

Conover, C.J. (2011, September 16). How private health insurance slashed the uninsured rate for Americans. Retrieved August 7, 2017 from: www.aei.org/publication /how-private-health-insurance-slashed-the-uninsured-rate-for-americans/

Eiken, S., Sredl, K., Burwell, B., & Gold, L. (2010, August 17). Medicaid long-term care expenditures in FY 2009. Retrieved from: www.nasuad.org/sites/nasuad/files /hcbs/files/193/9639/2009LTCExpenditures.pdf

Fisher, E.S., Staiger, D.O., Bynum, J.P.W., ...Gottlieb, D.J. (2007). Creating accountable care organizations: The extended hospital medical staff. *Health Affairs*, *21*(6), w44–w57. Retrieved July 2017 from: http://content.healthaffairs.org/content/26/1 /w44.abstract

Gleckman, H. (2012). What's killing the long-term-care insurance industry. *Forbes*. Retrieved December 1, 2017 from: www.forbes.com/sites/howardgleckman/2012/08 /29/what's-killing-the-long-term-care-insurance-industry

Harden, S. (2010). Six things you must know about never events. Life Wings. Retrieved July 2017 from: www.qprinstitute.com/pdfs/SixThingsYouNeed.pdf

Herman, B. (2016). Healthcare spending growth rate rises again in 2015. Retrieved July 2017 from: www.modernhealthcare.com/article/20160713/news/160719963

James, B.C., & Poulson, G.P. (2016, July-August). The case for capitation. *Harvard Business Review*. Retrieved from: https:/hbr.org/2016/07/the-case-for-capitation

Kaiser Family Foundation. (2016, September 14). 2016 employer health benefits survey. Retrieved August 7, 2017 from: www.kff.org/report-section/ehbs -2016-summary-of-findings/

McCall, N. (Ed.). (2001). *Who will pay for long-term care?* Chicago, IL: Health Administration Press.

Michael, C., & Chernew, E. (2003). Increased spending on health care: How much can the United States afford? *Health Affairs, 22*(4), 15. Retrieved July 2017 from: content.healthaffairs.org/content/22/4/15.full

Miller, H. (2007). *Creating payment systems to accelerate value-driven health care: Issues and options for policy reform.* New York: The Commonwealth Fund.

Ng, T., Harrington, C., & Kitchener, M. (2010). Medicare and Medicaid in long-term care. *Health Affairs, 29*(1), 22–28. Retrieved August 7, 2017 from: content.healthaf fairs.org/content/29/1/22.full

Oberlander, J. (2007). Learning from failure in health care reform. *New England Journal of Medicine, 357*, 1677–1679. doi: 10.1056/NEJMp078201

Paradise, J. (2014, July 17). The impact of the Children's Health Insurance Program (CHIP): What does the research tell us? Retrieved August 7, 2017 from: www.kff .org/medicaid/issue-brief/the-impact-of-the-childrens-health-insurance-program -chip-what-does-the-research-tell-us/

Physicians Foundation. (2016). 2016 survey of America's physicians: Practice patterns and perspectives. Retrieved August 7, 2017 from: www.physiciansfoundation.org /uploads/default/Biennial_Physician_Survey_2016.pdf

Rank, J. (2017). Employee health insurance—The history and economic theory of employer-provided health insurance. Retrieved December 1, 2017 from: medicine .rank.org/pages/561/Employee-Health-Insurance-history-economic=theory -employer-provided-health-insurance.html

Robinson, J., & Casalino, L. (1995). The growth of medical groups paid through capitation in California. *New England Journal of Medicine, 333*, 1684–1687.

Rosenberg, C.E. (1987). *The care of strangers: The rise of America's hospital system.* New York: Basic Books. Retrieved December 1, 2017 from: www.ncbi.nlm.nih.gov /pmcarticles/PMC4

Sharifi, H., & Zeydi, A. (2016). When is the best time to mobilize patients after myocardial infarction? An issue that merits further research. *Anatolian Journal of Cardiology, 16*, 547–552. doi: 10.14744/AnatolJCardiol.2016.7237

Tax Equity and Fiscal Responsibility Act of 1982. Public L. No: 97–248, 96 Stat. 324. (September 3, 1982). Retrieved from: www.congress.gov/bill/97th-congress /house-bill/4961

Thomas, S. (2013, January 7). The ACA and the responsibilities of the states. *Sanford Journal of Public Policy*. Retrieved July 2017 from: sites.duke.edu/sjpp/2013 /the-aca-and-responsibilities-of-the-states/

U.S. Department of Health & Human Services. (2005, January 24). Using Medicaid to support working-age adults with serious mental illnesses in the community. Retrieved August 7, 2017 from: https://aspe.hhs.gov/report/using-medicaid -support-working-age-adults-serious-mental-illnesses-community-handbook /brief-history-medicaid

U.S. Department of Health & Human Services. (2017, February 21). Medicare, Medicaid, and more. Retrieved July 2017 from: https://longtermcare.acl.gov /medicare-medicaid-more/

U.S. Department of Labor. (2017). Health plans and benefits: ERISA. Retrieved December 1, 2017 from: www.dol.gov/general/topic/health-plans/erisa

Part Three

Challenges in policy implementation

Examples from the field

6 Landscape for new models of care

Designing best practices and environments

I. Introduction

In the United States, those aged 65 and older are the fastest growing segment of the population, with numbers that will likely double in the next five decades, from 46 million in 2017 to projections of over 98 million by 2060 (U.S. Census Bureau, 2017). This rapid growth, coupled with continual advances in medical technology, will increase long-term-care spending and leave many older adults struggling to understand where they should live, what parts of their care are covered, and how to pay for gaps in services.

Older adults with functional limitations need assistance with housing, transportation, education, light housekeeping and meal preparation, personal assistance, and skilled nursing (Cox, 2005; Lynn, 2016). Aging well requires a wide range of services provided on an ongoing basis, while also effectively managing transitions as needs and health status change. With some exceptions, there is no set "formal system" or single point of entry for accessing these services. Even with this fragmentation, opportunities exist for meaningful collaboration between medical and non-medical providers, and several models have emerged.

The health care system and its ancillary services can be difficult to navigate at any age, but the complex needs of seniors in terms of maintaining independence while overcoming the barriers of declining functional capacity make it even more challenging for older Americans. Living longer poses physical, financial, and emotional challenges, compounded by the accompanying limitations on social interactions. A critical component of aging well is the need to stay connected with other people (Fowers, Richardson, & Slife, 2017); without meaningful social interaction, older adults develop feelings of loneliness and social isolation (Hawkley, Hughes, Waite, Masi, Thisted, & Cacioppo, 2008).

The public perception of aging creates common misconceptions regarding what aging well looks like; for the vast majority of people, significant existing gaps in services make it unlikely that those expectations will be met. Examining aging only through the lens of chronic disease and health status leads to massive lapses in understanding about what it means to grow old, akin to viewing the experience of childhood only through the lens of pediatrics. The challenge remains as to how to develop an elder-centered, community-based approach, which fosters independence while also providing resources and services for family caregivers. This is consistent with the World Health Organization's definition of health as "a state of complete physical, mental and social well being and not merely the absence of disease or infirmity" (World Health Organization, 2017). This repositioning towards a framework of overall health and quality of life is also necessary if we are to drive meaningful shifts in legislation, funding, and resources that will truly address the challenges our aging population faces.

As referenced in earlier chapters, literature and "scorecards" measuring success in aging services recommend that a high-performing system for long-term care supports and services must be coordinated with housing, transportation, and medical services, especially across settings during periods of transition (Reinhard et al., 2011). Several emerging initiatives and best practices focus on navigation among these varied public health considerations, either through traditional government structures, demonstration projects and pilot programs, or community-based nonprofits.

II.   Challenges in environment

A.   *Financial resources / Cost of care*

Providing appropriate quality services for older adults and meeting their needs across the continuum of care requires significant financial resources. With an aging population growing at historically unprecedented rates and ongoing cuts in Medicare and Medicaid reimbursements, the current structure is unsustainable. Older adults consume more health services than the general population. Meanwhile, 52% of this population in the United States has a chronic condition or functional limitation; providing care for this group represents 89% of U.S. health care costs (Institute of Medicine, 2015). Such services are not exclusively medical but include most long-term care, designating a range of services needed to meet personal care needs that are most often provided in the home, whether through community-based organizations or in long-term care facilities. The bulk of long-term care involves assisting people with activities of daily living, such as bathing and toilet use, dressing, transferring in and out of furniture, and eating. Other common task-oriented supports often help with "instrumental activities of daily living," which include housework, managing money, administering medication, meal preparation, and caring for pets (Cox, 2005). According to a survey of national costs by the insurance company Genworth (2017), the median cost for long-term care in the United States in 2016 was $6844 per month in a nursing home and $3628 per month in an assisted-living facility. Services for home health aides or homemakers were approximately $3861 per month, and services in an adult day care center cost about $1473 monthly. These numbers only represent the average costs of long-term care, as pricing depends on the setting, provider, and geographic location. Additionally, non-straightforward pricing leads to misunderstandings on the part of older adults and their families about what services and costs were covered, as compared to their assumptions. Understanding exactly what is covered is critical, especially at a younger age when proper planning can prevent higher costs later on (U.S. Department of Health & Human Services, 2017).

The major funders of long-term care are the Medicare and Medicaid programs, as delineated below (U.S. Department of Health & Human Services, 2017):

Medicare only pays for long-term care if skilled services or rehabilitative care are required:

- In a nursing home for a maximum of 100 days
- At home if receiving skilled home health or other skilled in-home services
- Skilled assistance with activities of daily living (ADLs) is not covered
- Recipient must pay for long-term care services that are not covered by a public or private insurance program

Medicaid pays for the largest share of long-term care services, but with income eligibility requirements:

- Income must be below a certain level and meet state eligibility requirements
- State eligibility requirements are based on the amount of assistance needed with ADLs
- Other federal programs such as the services provided through the Older Americans Act or Department of Veterans Affairs pay for long-term care services, but they have limits regarding specific populations or certain circumstances

B.   *Affordable senior housing*

Older adults struggle to find affordable and adequate housing, which constitutes a critical gap in aging services. While low-income seniors have some options available for subsidized housing, many live in inadequate, sometimes unsafe circumstances. Even older adults considered middle income struggle with housing and uncertain futures. Only those who meet the low-income requirements of Medicaid receive significant assistance for long-term care, with the result that many middle-class Americans are unable to afford these services out-of-pocket without financial supplementation (Houser, 2013). As aging, middle-income Baby Boomers face significant challenges in locating and paying for appropriate care, this largest generation in history must contemplate how to design their futures in ways that facilitate aging well while supplementing what Medicaid or Medicare covers.

Some older adults who have more financial resources opt for Continuing Care Retirement Communities (CCRCs), which allow them to live in one location for the remainder of their life with the option to move through various facilities within a single campus-like setting. CCRCs incorporate independent living, assisted living, and skilled nursing as options for older adults as they age. Healthy adults who sign up for continuing-care retirement communities can live independently in homes or condominiums until more assistance becomes necessary, at which time they can move to assisted living or nursing facilities. This continuum of care setting, while attractive, often comes with extremely expensive entrance fees and monthly charges. According to AARP, entrance fees to secure a spot can range from $100,000 to $1 million. Monthly charges range from $3000 to $5000, but these may also increase as needs change. Although CCRCs vary by community, basic services commonly include meals, grounds maintenance, local transportation, security systems, and on-site physician services. Some communities may offer more services, such as housekeeping, laundry service, or the processing of Medicare and insurance reimbursement forms (AARP, 2016).

C. Reliance on caregiving

The desire of older adults to remain in their homes as they age, coupled with shorter hospital stays and increased reliance on outpatient procedures, shifts more responsibility to informal caregivers (Alkema, 2013). Our health care system now relies heavily on unpaid or informal providers of care, transferring a tremendous burden onto family members who must assist with regular daily activities such as household tasks, driving loved ones to appointments, and often taking the lead on coordinating medical care (Arno, Levine, & Memmott, 1999). Some provide more intensive help with ADLs such as feeding, bathing, and administering medications. Family members often describe the emotional, physical, and financial toll of caring for a loved one.

This extra burden can lead to changes in family dynamics and conflict within families. The challenges of managing information-gathering, coordinating another person's needs, and making decisions can be overwhelming for caregivers and recipients, especially given the limited resources for support within our current system. In some areas, community-based organizations offer respite, information, and referrals for families, but these services do little to help with often overwhelming decision-making processes and navigation of complex health and human service systems. Long-distance caregiving, a necessity at a time when families are more spread apart, is even more onerous. In many cases, services are unavailable or not properly accessed, and costs are prohibitive. Caregivers often report strain on their physical health, emotional stress, and overwhelming financial burdens as a result of their role.

III. Programs and best practices

A. *Home and community-based services*

Many older adults receive care from family members and friends. As needs increase, this is supplemented with public or private agencies in their homes (Stone, 2011). For older adults, home-based providers represent an affordable way to remain at home longer while also meeting their needs for nutrition, medical care, socialization, home modifications, and other essentials (Weaver & Roberto, 2017). Challenges arise because services are not organized into an easily managed, systematic whole, owing to the piecemeal development of home- and community-based services, and the varying revenue streams. These providers, with functions and revenue sources that vary widely, are simply not designed for comprehensive home care.

The Federal Administration for Community Living (ACL), formed in 2012, strives for affordable and coordinated home- and community-based services that will help older adults remain at home, as designed by the Older Americans Act. The ACL works in conjunction with the Aging Services Network, a loose association of care providers in local communities, to develop a more coordinated system of home- and community-based long-term care. The aging network reaches approximately 11 million people each year, 3 million of whom receive more intensive services that include home-delivered meals, personal care, and homemaker services. Any senior aged 60 and older can seek services through the ACL, but the agency gives priority to low-income people with the greatest need (ACL, 2016).

These networks of local agencies aim to provide coordinated services for seniors. In many communities, senior centers serve as important resources connecting individuals with programs devoted to wellness, health screening, and self-care, which can be critical for those who wish to remain in their homes. They also offer opportunities for social connections and coordination where additional assistance is needed. In the continuum of long-term care, such centers offer a less formal means of accessing necessary supports while giving seniors the freedom to come and go as they please. Other community resources like adult day services provide structured social programs, recreation, and support services for older adults who require more care and supervision than a senior center traditionally offers. Day programs allow older adults who might otherwise require residential care to continue living at home. Such services also provide support and respite for family caregivers, and in particular, assure family caregivers who hold other jobs that their older relative will receive both supervision and social engagement during their working hours.

Senior centers and day programs provide older adults with opportunities for services and supports in settings where they feel safe and comfortable (Cox, 2005). A telehealth program in Westchester County, New York inspired by this concept has gained attention for its innovations. Telehealth Intervention Programs for Seniors (TIPS) is a community-embedded, remote patient monitoring service for seniors. It combines three key elements: clinical monitoring of vital signs (blood pressure, pulse, oxygen levels, and weight), a social check-in to make sure seniors are aware of all the ancillary support services (nutrition, transportation, caregiving, etc.), and intergenerational interactions between seniors and students from local colleges. Local college students, following the completion of some basic training, visit senior sites and transmit data to graduate student nurses who review it remotely. Student nurses will contact the seniors, their caregivers or primary care physicians directly if any of the vitals show cause for concern. Seniors receive a comprehensive assessment that includes an explanation of their tests and recommendations for additional services. While telehealth programs are increasingly becoming trusted tools, TIPS also integrates social supports through its Livable Communities Initiative. The program is funded by Westchester's Department of Senior Programs and Services, the Harry and Jeannette Weinberg Foundation, and the Public/Private Partnership for Aging.

A federal initiative, the Program of All-Inclusive Care for the Elderly (PACE), provides long-term services and supports to Medicaid and Medicare enrollees (approximately 40,000) who are at risk of institutionalization to help them remain in their homes. Using an interdisciplinary team of health professionals, PACE integrates a range of social supports. The program's financing structure allows participants to obtain all services they need that are offered within the model, not just those that are reimbursable under Medicare and Medicaid. Individuals must be 55 or older, live in the service area of a PACE organization, qualify for nursing home care, and be able to live safely in the community (Cox, 2005). Benefits include any services deemed necessary, including primary care, hospital care, medical specialty services, prescription drugs, home care, physical and occupational therapy, adult day care, recreational therapy, meals, nutritional counseling, social services, social work counseling, and transportation. Although often criticized for its restrictions in choosing providers, PACE exemplifies a model of all-inclusive care that incorporates social supports, transportation, and medical services, and demonstrates how public policy support of coordinated services aimed at fulfilling the needs of the whole person can be viable (Lynn, 2016).

B.   The aging in place movement

Older adults are moving beyond rigid notions of biomedical care delivered in traditional medical settings to embrace broader concepts, including desirable and affordable alternatives for receiving care in the home. Recent public policy changes, referenced previously, support a transition from a health care system that views institutional settings as the default to one that encourages "aging in place." No such coordinated effort exists for older Americans, making this a key policy priority at a time when institutionalization remains the norm rather than the exception. Older Americans express a widespread desire to remain at home, and community-based care has been shown to be less costly than institutional care (Marek, Stetzer, Adams, Popejoy, & Rantz, 2012). These aging-in-place alternatives warrant consideration among lawmakers and regulators for their potential to help older adults age successfully in the community (Scharlach, 2017).

Another approach, known as the village model, offers great promise. Community-based membership organizations, called villages, offer activities and supportive services for older adults who wish to remain at home. In exchange for a fee of a few hundred dollars per year on average, members receive help with shopping, house maintenance, transportation, referrals to vetted home care professionals, and medical and care-management services. The network of resources and activities in villages revolve around both daily living needs and deeper personal fulfillment, acknowledging social, cultural, and health and wellness dimensions. Village personnel direct members to vetted providers after negotiating discounted rates and connect members to volunteers who help with a range of services. Villages describe their mission as the enhancement of members' lives by facilitating social connections and support services, which in turn enables people to enjoy a richness of experience, personal independence, and a healthy quality of life. They function to provide a trusted source for information and referrals within their communities. As of 2017, 85 member-based neighborhood networks—villages—were operating in the country, and about 140 were in development. By creating aging-friendly communities that work in conjunction with community services, villages bring together groups of older Americans as a loose but vital association of neighbors, rather than just "housing" people (Scharlach, 2017). Boston's Beacon Hill Village, started in 2002, was the first to establish the initial village concept and is still considered the best known. Overall, these models have gained popularity for their potential to help older Americans, including middle-class ones, age in their communities.

Although each village reflects the needs of its own unique community, they all share certain hallmark characteristics, according to the Village to Village Network:

- Structured as self-governing, self-supporting, grassroots membership-based organizations
- Offer consolidation and coordination of services to members
- Create new partnerships that leverage existing community resources, not duplicating existing services
- Follow a holistic, person-centered, member-driven ethos
- Promote volunteerism, civic engagement, and intergenerational connections (Village to Village Network, 2017).

The integration of social and medical supports and the coordination between silos, regardless of funding streams, represent the most intriguing features of this model. While some opportunities of this nature exist within current policies, they are limited in scope and availability. Given their current composition (most are middle class), and the limited research supporting the value of social supports, villages will continue to struggle to fit into current public policy discussions.

Naturally occurring retirement communities (NORCs), often referenced in aging-in-place discussions, developed in the context of dense locations, such as apartment buildings, that can accommodate services and supports in a relatively central place. This "naturally occurring" concept captured the attention of aging experts as a promising model for supporting older adults in their own environments, and many states have some variation of NORC-specific supportive services programs (Greenfield, 2016). The United Hospital Fund, a health-care-oriented nonprofit, developed a NORC blueprint website to help communities replicate these programs across the country. The characteristics of a NORC vary, but generally include a minimum concentration of seniors and minimum age of entry ranging from 50 to 65 years old within a specific geographic area. Examples of the types of services provided by a NORC-focused program include case management, home care, transportation, meals, social and cultural events, health care management and preventative activities, mental health services, bereavement support, and exercise classes, among many others. Funding flows from a mix of public and private sources.

AARP's Livable Community Initiative strives to help cities and towns create built environments that allow older adults to thrive with relative independence, such as walkable streets, accessible public transportation, and opportunities to engage in social and civic life. While the concept of making cities more livable may benefit older people in particular, such traits make them more livable for everyone. Because livable communities also attract younger people, a "neighbor-helping-neighbor" philosophy can take root that features volunteer programs for younger people to assist older adults in need of help (AARP, 2016).

Another model, popularized by The Robert Wood Johnson Foundation's National Volunteer Caregiving Network (NVCN), gives congregations opportunities for volunteering to help seniors remain independent. Originally called Faith in Action from its 1983 inception through 2008, NVCN works through a network of hundreds of autonomous programs, offering free services to anyone who needs them. Similar to the village model, each NVCN member program is unique but they all share common principles: interfaith traditions, the use volunteers, and caregiving that focuses on daily tasks such as transportation, errands, respite for caregivers, and light housekeeping (NCVN, 2017). Also like the village model, the parent organization relies on the leadership of a paid coalition director who reports to a volunteer board, working to carry out principles under a strong citizen-led philosophy. (See Appendix D, Resources and Program Examples for Older Adults for additional resource information on program models.)

All of these models share some of the same core concepts. They all provide a range of services and while not always offering them directly, coordinate and facilitate those services for members. Citizen-led, volunteer-driven initiatives such as NORC and NCVN work to offer social supports through a neighbor-helping-neighbor philosophy. The significant contributions of volunteer-based services speak to the importance of fulfilling the non-medical ancillary needs of older Americans who would like to remain in their homes. In addition to being cost-effective, tapping into a volunteer base offers opportunities for strong social connections among community members (Fowers et al., 2017). Given the increase in the older adult population, expense of traditional long-term care services, and precariousness of funding, innovative solutions like the ones seen in these models are critical.

C. *The integration of medical and social supports*

Aging in place is desirable for various reasons, yet without proper supports to accompany this, isolation may result that in turn leads to physical and emotional vulnerability and inadequate health care. The higher prevalence of disease and disability in older adults leads them to consume more health care, and experience limitations that adversely affect their treatment and recovery (Longest, 2015). The gradual decline in activities of daily living that is typical of seniors makes a healthy lifestyle difficult to maintain. Changes in health status often happen rapidly, especially when other serious health conditions are present such as heart disease or diabetes. The effects of disease further complicate the emotional and practical concerns of older adults, which in turn affects how they cope with their illness. The toll of social isolation and reliance on family and friends, coupled with fears over the costs of their care, can overwhelm older adults and their caregivers. Large health systems and community-based services often face the same challenge of how to keep older adults healthy and safe after discharge from a hospital stay, or while receiving health services in the home (Lynn, 2016).

The challenge of person-centered cancer care:
Shift to elder-centered care

The steady increase in cancer diagnoses—a disease that disproportionately affects older adults—necessitates models that integrate medical services with social supports. More than 13.7 million cancer survivors live in the United States today, and more than 1.5 million people receive new diagnoses each year (American Cancer Society, 2017). The last several years have seen substantial progress in cancer treatments, resulting in both increased life expectancy and a new dynamic of people living with cancer as a chronic illness. Although these individuals face complex decisions related to their care, from treatment choices to financial options for coverage, less than one-third of people facing cancer receive appropriate counseling and support. A 2008 Institute of Medicine committee noted:

> The remarkable advances in biomedical care for cancer have not been matched by achievements in providing high-quality care for the psychological and social effects of cancer. Numerous cancer survivors and their caregivers report that cancer care providers did not understand their psychosocial needs, failed to recognize and adequately address depression and other symptoms of stress, were unaware of or did not refer them to available resources, and generally did not consider psychosocial support to be an integral part of quality cancer care.
>
> (Institute of Medicine, 2008)

In the last several years since that landmark Institute of Medicine (IOM) report, *Cancer Care for the Whole Patient: Meeting Psychosocial Health Needs*, awareness of the value of psychosocial support has grown. A number of other organizations have recognized the importance of social and emotional care in their quality recommendations, including the Patient-Center Outcomes Research Institute (PCORI): 2012 Research Agenda, American College of Surgeons Commission on Cancer: 2012 Patient-Centered Standards, American Society of Clinical Oncology: Quality Oncology Practice Initiative (QOPI), and Community Oncology Alliance: Oncology Medical Home.

The Institute of Medicine report defines psychosocial health services as "psychological and social services and interventions that enable patients, their families, and health care providers to optimize biomedical health care and to manage the psychological/behavioral and social aspects of illness and its consequences so as to promote better health" (Institute of Medicine, 2008). People who live in community-based settings have long understood the value of this emotional and social support. Navigating the ever-changing emotional terrain that accompanies cancer can be difficult, even when surrounded by supportive family and friends. Whether receiving a diagnosis, undergoing treatment, or recovering post-treatment, the right emotional supports are an essential complement to medical care. Psychosocial stress can emerge from any number of factors, including fears about death, side effects of disease and treatment, lack of education about what to expect, transportation issues, concern for how loved ones are coping, and financial anxieties, whether concerning health insurance payments, household bills, or fear of the future costs of treatments.

While the health care community increasingly understands the importance of addressing patients' psychological and social needs for quality care and better health, more progress is necessary to spread awareness of that concept and integrate it as a standard practice. The IOM report and other landmark studies have validated psychosocial support, demonstrating the need for traditional medical cancer care to fully integrate these services as fundamental components of treatment. In their article "A New Quality Standard: The Integration of Psychosocial Care into Routine Cancer Care," Jacobsen and

Wagner examined findings in several studies that identified harmful effects to patients with unmet psychosocial needs and found evidence that patients greatly benefited from psychosocial services. Despite this evidence, they found current data suggest that a considerable portion of the population of those with cancer do not receive psychosocial care:

> Three lines of professional activity initiated in recent years have the potential to address this issue in fundamental ways: the formulation of standards of cancer care that address the psychosocial component of care, the issuance of clinical practice guidelines for psychosocial care of patients with cancer, and the development and implementation of measurable indicators of the quality of psychosocial care in oncology settings.
>
> (Jacobsen & Wagner, 2012)

Other similar findings show that depression reduces the ability of patients with chronic disease to adhere to medical regimens (Katon, 2011). Still others show that psychosocial interventions improve health outcomes and survival rates (Andersen et al., 2007), as well as reduce emotional distress, anxiety, and depression, and raise health-related quality of life (Faller et al., 2013) with reduced recurrence and death (Andersen et al., 2008). (See Appendix C, Psychosocial Support, for additional resource information on psychosocial support services.)

D.   Enhancing collaboration and communication

A partnership between an organization that offers support to people with cancer and the medical teams treating those patients

In community settings, patients and their families often struggle to receive the supportive services necessary to fulfill their biopsychosocial needs. As patients seek support in disparate settings, new models of care delivery have begun integrating support services from community-based agencies. The WESTMED Medical Group and Gilda's Club Westchester (GCW), both located in Westchester County, New York, developed a partnership that integrates community-based oncology and palliative care with programs for individuals with cancer that focus on emotional and social dimensions.

Gilda's Club Westchester offers psychosocial support for individuals with cancer, along with their caregivers and family members. Specific services include: individual counseling, family counseling, survivorship and coping skills programs, and support groups that are organized by diagnosis, such as breast or lung cancer, or by circumstance, such as recently diagnosed, in treatment, or post-treatment. All services are offered free of charge and specialized to meet the needs of men, women, children and teens, and caregivers. WESTMED Medical Group, an integrated practice of more than 500 physicians and 1200 clinical employees, provides comprehensive care that focuses on quality of life and on reducing suffering at any stage of illness.

These organizations work in concert to treat the whole person throughout the course of their cancer experience.

In an era of person-centered care, the quality of care depends on health care teams sharing knowledge and information. Recognizing this fact, clinicians from WESTMED and GCW closely collaborate and communicate to better support patients and their family members.

At the heart of this partnership are methods for addressing some of the most fundamental questions about how to provide quality care:

- What barriers impede cross-functional communications and hinder knowledge-sharing among separate organizations?
- How can professionals in these separate community-based settings enhance their communication with one another?
- What barriers deter access to and utilization of oncology and palliative care and psychosocial services?

The partnership aims to blend the approaches of different sets of providers into a single team, whereby WESTMED refers patients to Gilda's Club, which in turn loops in the WESTMED medical team regarding patients' psychosocial status. Oncology and palliative care patients receive a formal referral to Gilda's Club generated through an electronic medical record. Gilda's staff are integrated onsite at WESTMED, offering various programs at medical facilities while familiarizing patients with the nearby Gilda's facility as an approachable place to receive additional supportive services. In addition to providing individual counseling, Gilda's Club offers specialized programs onsite that include a survivorship series to address emotional challenges in the post-treatment phase, and a coping skills series. These time-limited, didactic trainings have shown significant promise for alleviating the stress and anxiety that often accompany a cancer diagnosis while providing tools for coping. Social workers also attend clinical meetings at WESTMED in order to integrate psychosocial needs of patients into their care plans and infuse a culture of emotional and social support for patients and their families.

IV.   Conclusion

Given that aging well requires a coordinated system that incorporates both medical and non-medical supports, innovative models have been integrating a number of supports across disciplines. These models show promise in how they conceive care and address the challenges that older adults and their caregivers must negotiate. Many of the more successful programs are being replicated in additional communities across the United States, but still struggle with sustainability and funding concerns. Collaboration between providers holds the key to the future of care, and leaders must proceed with that spirit of collaboration as a guiding principle. Meaningful partnerships among providers currently operating under different models may offer opportunities for higher-quality care and prospects to address gaps in services. As these models continue to gain momentum and show positive outcomes, coupled with their potential to lower costs, they may inform policy discussions going forward.

References

AARP Livable Communities. (2016). What is a livable community? Retrieved December 2016 from: www.aarp.org/livable-communities/about/info-2014/what-is -a-livable-community.html

Alkema, G.E. (2013, March). Current issues and potential solutions for addressing America's long-term care financing crisis. Retrieved from: www.thescanfounda tion.org/sites/default/files/tsf_ltc-financing_overview_alkema_3-20-13.pdf

American Cancer Society. (2017). *Cancer facts & figures 2017*. Atlanta, GA: American Cancer Society. Retrieved from: www.cancer.org/content/dam/cancer-org/research /cancer-facts-and-statistics/annual-cancer-facts-and-figures/2017/cancer-facts-and -figures-2017.pdf

Andersen, B.L., Farrar, W.B., Golden-Kreutz, D., Emery, C.F., Glaser, R., Crespin, T., & Carson, W.E. (2007). Distress reduction from a psychological intervention contributes to improved health for cancer patients. *Brain, Behavior, and Immunity*, *21*(7), 953–961. http://doi.org/10.1016/j.bbi.2007.03.005

Andersen, B.L., Yang, H.C., Farrar, W.B., Golden-Kreutz, D.M., Emery, C.F., Thornton, L.M., … Carson, W.E. (2008). Psychologic intervention improves survival for breast cancer patients. *Cancer*, *113*(12), 3450–3458.

Arno, P., Levine, C., & Memmott, M.M. (1999). The economic value of informal care-giving. *Health Affairs*, *18*(2), 182–188. doi:10.1377/hlthaff.18.2.182

Cox, C.B. (2005). *Community care for an aging society: Issues, policies, and services*. New York: Springer.

Faller, H., Schuler, M., Richard, M., Heckl, U., Weis, J., & Kuffner, R. (2013). Effects of psycho-oncologic interventions on emotional distress and quality of life in adult patients with cancer: systematic review and meta-analysis. *Journal of Clinical Oncology. 31*, 782–793.

Fowers, B., Richardson, F., & Slife, B. (2017). *Frailty, suffering, and vice: Flourishing in the face of human limitations*. Washington, DC: American Psychological Association.

Genworth Financial, Inc. (2017, August 14). Cost of care survey 2017. Retrieved from: www.genworth.com/about-us/industry-expertise/cost-of-care.html

Greenfield, E.A. (2016). Support from neighbors and aging in place: Can NORC programs make a difference? *Gerontologist*, *56*(4), 651–659.

Hawkley, L.C., Hughes, M.E., Waite, L.J., Masi, C.M., Thisted, R.A., & Cacioppo, J.T. (2008). From social structural factors to perceptions of relationship quality and loneliness: The Chicago Health, Aging, and Social Relations Study. *Journals of Gerontology. Series B, Psychological Sciences and Social Sciences*, *63*(6), S375–S384.

Houser, A. (2013). *A new way of looking at private pay affordability of long-term services and supports*. Washington, DC: AARP Public Policy Institute.

Institute of Medicine (IOM). (2008). *Cancer care for the whole patient: Meeting psychosocial health needs*. Washington, DC: National Academies Press.

Institute of Medicine (IOM). (2015). *Dying in America: Improving quality and honoring individual preferences near the end of life*. Washington, DC: National Academies Press. doi: 10.17226/18748

Jacobsen, P.B., & Wagner, L.I. (2012). A new quality standard: The integration of psycho-social care into routine cancer care. *Journal of Clinical Oncology, 30*(11), 1154–1159.

Katon, W. (2011). Epidemiology and treatment of depression in patients with chronic medical illness. *Dialogues in Clinical Neuroscience, 13*(1), 7–23.

Longest, B. (2015). *Health policymaking in the United States.* Chicago, IL: Health Administration Press.

Lynn, J. (2016). *MediCaring communities: Getting what we want and need in frail old age at an affordable cost.* Altarum Institute.

Marek, K., Stetzer, F., Adams, S., Popejoy, L., & Rantz, M. (2012). Aging in place versus nursing home care: Comparison of costs to Medicare and Medicaid. *Research in Gerontological Nursing, 5*(2), 123–129. doi: 10.3928/19404921-20110802-01

National Volunteer Caregiving Network (NVCN). A history of volunteer caregiving. Retrieved October 2017 from: www.nvcnetwork.org/index.php/about-us/history

Naturally Occurring Retirement Communities (NORC) Programs. (2015). NORC blueprint: A guide to community action. Retrieved December 2017 from: www .norcblueprint.org

Older Americans Act of 1965, 42 U.S.C. §3025(a)(2)(E).

Reinhard, S.C, Kassner, E., Houser, A., & Mollica, R. (2011, September). Raising expectations: A state scorecard on long-term services and supports for older adults, people with physical disabilities, and family caregivers. Retrieved from: https:// assets.aarp.org/rgcenter/ppi/ltc/ltss_scorecard.pdf

Scharlach, A. (2017). Aging in context: Individual and environmental pathways to aging-friendly communities—The 2015 Matthew A. Pollack Award lecture. *Gerontologist, 57*(4), 606–618.

Stone, R. (2011). *Long-term care for the elderly.* Washington, DC: Urban Institute Press.

U.S. Census Bureau. (2017). U.S. population projections: 2014-2060. Retrieved from: www.census.gov/ population/projections/data/national/2014.html

U.S. Department of Health & Human Services. Medicare. Retrieved January 2017 from: https://longtermcare.acl.gov/medicare-medicaid-more/medicare.html

Village to Village Network. Village model. Retrieved December 2016 from: http:// vtvnetwork.org/content.aspx?page_id=22&club_id=691012&module_id=248578

Weaver, R.H., & Roberto, K.H. (2017). Home and community-based service use by vulnerable adults. *Gerontologist, 57*(3), 540–551.

World Health Organization. Preamble to the Constitution of WHO as adopted by the International Health Conference, New York, 19 June–22 July 1946; signed on 22 July 1946 by the representatives of 61 States (Official Records of WHO, no. 2, p. 100) and entered into force on 7 April 1948.

Bibliography

Carlson, L.E., & Bultz, B.D. (2004). Efficacy and medical cost offset of psycho-social interventions in cancer care: Making the case for economic analyses. *Psychooncology, 13*(12), 837–849.

Scharlach, A., Lehning, A., & Graham, C. (2010). *A demographic profile of village members.* Berkeley: University of California, Berkeley, Center for Advanced Study of Aging Services.

World Health Organization (WHO). (2006, October). *Constitution of the World Health Organization—Basic documents.* (45th ed., Supplement). Geneva, Switzerland: World Health Organization.

7 The palliative turn in elder-centered care

A public health strategy for interdisciplinary palliative and end-of-life care

I. Introduction

The twenty-first century will likely be the century of palliative care in aging and public health. Although the *Lancet* Commission (Knaul et al., 2017) has declared a global "access abyss" in palliative care and pain relief, the United States, as a high-income country, is seeing measured progress in the growth of palliative care across the care continuum—but a great deal more progress needs to be made. We frame palliative care, which encompasses hospice and end-of-life care as among its subsets (Jennings, Ryndes, D'Onofrio, & Baily, 2003), as a public health response to suffering, and more specifically for the purposes of this chapter, the suffering of older persons. The direction in palliative care is towards population health management and design of population-level interventions, including community-based primary care, that will mitigate suffering and improve quality of life. The shift from palliative medicine to palliative systems of care that integrate specialized medical care and socially directed supportive care (Morrissey, Herr, & Levine, 2015) will be key to the future of U.S. health care, especially for older persons.

One of the biggest challenges today for older persons when they encounter frailty, limitations, and serious illness is understanding the meaning of care and its diverse contexts—personal, family, systems, medical, social, and cultural. Some of the questions that come to mind about elder care, for both older adults and the persons who serve them in the aging and health systems, include:

- What is the culture or ethos of palliative and end-of-life care for older adults?
- Do older adults have human rights that must be honored in the provision of palliative and end-of-life care?
- What types of palliative and end-of-life care are available to older adults, and how and where can older adults access the care they need?
- What do best practices in palliative and end-of-life care look like?
- What policy- and systems-level changes need to be addressed to afford equitable access to palliative care and pain relief?

These are among the questions we examine in this chapter in advancing what we call a *palliative turn* in elder-centered care, that is, the embedding of the palliative approach to care across all levels of aging and health systems and the society—from hospital to community. This is a goal that is in full harmony with a public health strategy for palliative care as developed and advanced by the World Health Organization (Stjernswärd, Foley, & Ferris, 2007), and the well-recognized human right to health (United Nations, 1948; Sen, 2008; Wronka, 2008; Gostin, 2014).

II.   Health and human rights framework: The right to health

In the realm of aging and public health, we situate palliative care at the nexus of health and human rights, such as human rights to water and sanitation, food, housing, education, and transportation. In the early 1990s, Jonathan Mann and colleagues (1994) recognized this relationship and described its mutual and interdependent character: health, itself a human right, could act to support and re-enforce other human rights, or marginalization of the right to health through health policy making could interfere with the full attainment of such other human rights. Conversely, burdens on human rights or human rights violations could compromise achievement of health. Thus, health is not constituted in medical facilities and health delivery systems alone, but rather in and through environmental conditions and modifications of such conditions as would support the fundamental right to health—including older persons' right to health.

One of the most powerful examples of the interaction between the right to health—including the right to palliative care and pain relief, and human rights may be seen in the relationship between education and health. Findings from a nationwide study conducted in Belgium suggest that differences in individual educational levels influence access to specialist-level palliative care services and general practitioner contacts at the end of life (Bossuyt et al., 2011). Olshansky and colleagues (2012) report on the impact of race and education on life expectancy in the United States and identify an education-health-longevity gradient, as well as widening gaps in life expectancy demarcated by educational level and racial group membership. Mather, Jacobson, and Pollard (2015) have linked low educational attainment or fewer years of education among older women to lower income and poverty levels. Low health and financial literacy can also be a significant barrier to decision making. This body of evidence has important implications for meaningful participation in the health systems and the exercise of autonomy and self-determination.

In 2000, the United Nations Committee on Economic, Social and Cultural Rights adopted General Comment No. 14 (Committee on Economic, Social and Cultural Rights), recognizing the right to health as enjoyment of the highest attainable standard of health. General Comment No. 14 provides authoritative guidance on the right to health. As spelled out in the "Report of the Special Rapporteur" on the right of everyone to the enjoyment of the highest attainable standard of physical and mental health (Hunt, 2007), the right to health, which is broader than "health care," is understood as, "a right to an effective and integrated health system, encompassing health care and the underlying determinants of health, which is responsive to national and local priorities, and accessible to all" (p. 2). The right to health requires a two-fold assurance of entitlements and freedoms: assurances of effective and accessible health systems; and the right to freedom from interference such as torture or non-consensual medical treatment and experimentation (United Nations Office of the High Commissioner for Human Rights, 2008).

A. The right to palliative care and pain relief

According to General Comment No. 14, the normative content of the right to health comprises availability, accessibility, ethical and cultural acceptability, quality and the non-discriminatory provision of health facilities, goods and services (Gostin, 2014). This normative right to health is inclusive of rights to palliative care *and* pain management. In *The Global Palliative Care Atlas* (Connor & Sepulveda, 2014), the authors clarify that while General Comment No. 14 contains no express reference to palliative care, the Comment explicates the normative content of the right to health, including access to essential medicines, and specifies the core obligations of all signatory nations without regard to nations' resources, "These obligations include access to health facilities, provision of goods and services on a nondiscriminatory basis, the provision of essential medicines as defined by the WHO, and the adoption and implementation of a public health strategy" (Connor & Sepulveda, 2014, p. 9). States' obligation to operationalize the right to health under international law is also not expunged by the absence of a constitutional right to health care, such as in the United States. The UN Special Rapporteur on torture has recognized that "denying access to pain relief can amount to inhuman and degrading treatment" (Connor & Sepulveda, 2014, p. 9).

In 2010, delegates to the International Pain Summit of the International Association for the Study of Pain voted to support the Montreal Declaration (IASP, 2010), a policy statement explicitly declaring and recognizing the right to pain management as a fundamental human right.

III. International palliative care frameworks and recommendations

A. WHO Public Health Strategy for Palliative Care

The Public Health Strategy (PHS) for Palliative Care advances a robust agenda for translating knowledge, evidence, and innovation into effective population-level interventions and practices for relieving suffering and improving quality of life for persons with illness and serious illness across the life span. The PHS encompasses four key components:

- Formulation of national policies and regulations, including development of funding sources and service delivery models.
- Assurance of adequate drug availability, including access to essential medicines such as opioids, and addressing costs, prescribing, distribution, dispensing, and administration.
- Provision of education and training for all health care and community health workers and members of the public.
- Effective implementation of policy through strategic business plans, infrastructure, standards, and guidelines (Stjernswärd, Foley, & Ferris, 2007, p. 491).

"Palliative care for all" (Stjernswärd, Foley, & Ferris, 2007, p. 491) or palliative care everywhere, including palliative care experts, health care professionals, and the community—also described as "palliative environments" by Morrissey, Herr, and Levine (2015)—is integral to the last phase of the strategy—policy implementation.

B.   WHO definition of palliative care

The WHO definition of palliative care frames the goals of the palliative approach and provides a comprehensive description of palliative care services:

Palliative care is an approach that improves the quality of life of patients and their families facing the problem associated with life-threatening illness, through the prevention and relief of suffering by means of early identification and impeccable assessment and treatment of pain and other problems, physical, psychosocial and spiritual. Palliative care:

- provides relief from pain and other distressing symptoms;
- affirms life and regards dying as a normal process;
- intends neither to hasten or postpone death;
- integrates the psychological and spiritual aspects of patient care;
- offers a support system to help patients live as actively as possible until death;
- offers a support system to help the family cope during the patient's illness and in their own bereavement;
- uses a team approach to address the needs of patients and their families, including bereavement counselling, if indicated;
- will enhance quality of life, and may also positively influence the course of illness;

- is applicable early in the course of illness, in conjunction with other therapies that are intended to prolong life, such as chemotherapy or radiation therapy, and includes those investigations needed to better understand and manage distressing clinical complications.

(World Health Organization, n.d.; Connor and Sepulveda, 2014)

The *Lancet* Commission (2017) has cited both the strengths and limitations of the WHO definition, using it as a starting point but recommending that it be reviewed and revised to remove any reference to time or prognostication limits on access to palliative care, and to take account of health system levels and advances, and low income as well as other settings.

C. *67th World Health Assembly Resolution on Palliative Care*

Most recently, at the 67th World Health Assembly, the WHO adopted a Resolution (WHA 67.19), calling for "Strengthening of palliative care as a component of comprehensive care throughout the life course" (World Health Organization, 2014). WHO's Ad Hoc Technical Advisory Panel on Palliative Care is overseeing implementation of the palliative care resolution and as part of that process, has developed *a Guide for Programme Managers* (2016) (hereinafter "Manual") that provides a blueprint for mapping out and implementing palliative care programs and best practices on the ground. The Manual expands on the WHO definition of palliative care:

> Palliative care is the prevention and relief of suffering of any kind—physical, psychological, social, or spiritual—experienced by adults and children living with life-limiting health problems. It promotes dignity, quality of life and adjustment to progressive illnesses, using best available evidence ... All people, irrespective of income, disease type, or age, should have access to a nationally determined set of basic health services, including palliative care. Financial and social protection systems need to take into account the human right to palliative care for poor and marginalized population groups.
>
> (World Health Organization, 2016, p. 5)

In Building Integrated Palliative Care Programs and Services (2017), the authors also identify the following principles and values of Palliative Care Public Health Programs grounded in recognition of palliative care as a human right:

- Support to persons suffering in vulnerable conditions, with respect for their values and preferences;
- Universal coverage, equity, access and quality to every patient in need of it;

- Population-based, community oriented, integrated into the health care system and into the culture;
- Model of care: based on patients and families' needs and demands, respectful, patient and family-centered;
- Model of organisation: based on competent interdisciplinary teams, with clinical ethics, integrated care, case management, and advance care planning;
- Quality: effectiveness, efficiency, satisfaction, continuity, sustainability;
- Evidence-based, systematic evaluation of results, accountability;
- Social interaction and involvement; and
- Innovation in the organization of the Health Care System.

(World Health Organization, 2017, p. 66)

D.   Lancet Commission Report on Palliative Care

In a groundbreaking and visionary report on palliative care, The *Lancet* Commission (2017) decries the moral failing of the global public health systems in the face of extreme suffering, unrelieved pain, poverty and inequity across the world, especially in low- and middle-income countries. The Commission calls for worldwide recognition of palliative care and pain relief as essential components of universal health coverage and social provision, and progressive realization of these goals. Tracing the modern history of palliative care that emerged in the 1960s and 1970s, as well as its nineteenth-century roots in the first articulated principles of palliative medicine—including Munk's recognized 1887 treatise on death in which he describes the need for practical, spiritual and medical end-of-life support, the Commission cites important milestones as summarized below:

PANEL 3: A HISTORY OF PALLIATIVE CARE

Modern palliative care emerged in the 1960s and 1970s, though with much earlier roots. In the nineteenth century, doctors devised the principles of palliative medicine showing the value of new pain-relieving medicines and technologies and mapping the challenges of caring for those with advanced disease at a time when society became concerned about the process of dying. Notable was Munk's 1887 treatise on easeful death, in which he described practical, spiritual, and medical end-of-life support.

In parallel, specialized institutional care for dying people in hospices began in several countries, including France, Great Britain, India, South Africa, the United States and Zimbabwe. Although limited in scale, their philosophy of care inspired others.

Among them was Cicely Saunders who launched a movement in the 1960s for care of the dying, incorporating new knowledge and methods. Her concept of total pain with physical, social, psychological, and spiritual dimensions, revolutionized thinking and practice. She offered a positive, imaginative alternative to medicine's despairing rejection of dying patients and sought to ensure pain relief, maintain dignity, and enhance remaining life, however short. Her approach was embodied in St. Christopher's Hospice, founded in 1967 as the first modern hospice to include research and training facilities. Its influence quickly spread worldwide.

To gain traction in the word of medicine, these protagonists moved from activism to a concerted body of knowledge and practice. Management of cancer pain proved key. Early studies explored and reconsidered prevailing orthodoxies. New competence emerged in use of morphine and other medicines, reinforced by clinical research, which fueled investment and growth in services.

Balfour Mount is credited with coining palliative care, a term adopted in the 1970s that came to signify the transfer of hospice principles into wider settings within the health-care system, including acute care hospitals, primary care, and homes. Specialist journals were created to disseminate research and clinical practice, and national and international associations were formed. A new field of research was created.

Formal recognition of palliative medicine as a specialty began in the UK in 1987 and extended to other countries and to nursing. WHO had a major role in 1986 when it acknowledged the undertreatment of cancer pain as a public health problem and published the revolutionary "pain relief ladder" with simple recommendations to treat pain in three steps: mild, moderate, and severe. Recognizing the need for a comprehensive approach to palliative care, WHO published a definition of palliative care in 1990 and emphasized the importance of symptom management and pain relief. In a 2002 revision, WHO extended their definition of palliative care beyond cancer.

The field of palliative care was now poised for a global role, and high levels of unmet need were identified. Palliative care was drawn increasingly to a public health framework of appropriate policies, services, and interventions, together with suitable quality assurance and evaliation. Full recognition of the opportunities and challenges came with the World Health Assembly Resolution of 2014 calling all governments to integrate plans for palliative care into their national health policies.

(Knaul et al., 2017, p. 9)

**PANEL 16: AN ESSENTIAL PACKAGE OF
RESOURCES AND INTERVENTIONS TO RESPOND
TO THE BURDEN OF SERIOUS HEALTH-RELATED
SUFFERING: KEY RECOMMENDATIONS**

- All countries should ensure universal access to an Essential Package by 2030.
- This Essential Package should be publicly financed for all families that could face financial catastrophe or impoverishment.
- Basic social supports should complement this package and be financed over and above the health budget, in coordination with social welfare programs.
- Policies and additional investment must be in place to ensure safe supply chains, to train and build up necessary human resources with an approach based on competencies in palliative care, and to avoid pressure to include costly formulations of pain medication.
- Access to best international pricing for medicines, especially inexpensive, off-patent injectable, and oral immediate-release morphine, is a priority for achieving universal coverage of the Essential Package.
- All efforts to expand access to best prices and to reduce costs of pain medicines should be complemented with technical assistance to ensure safe supply chains and medical use.
- Countries should develop a palliative care and pain relief package for children, taking special account of their specific social and spiritual needs.
- UNICEF can take the lead in establishing a special US$1 million annual fund for children living in low-income countries who are in need of opioids for the relief of pain and palliative care.

(Knaul et al., 2017, p. 37)

The *Lancet* Commission Report is focused primarily on palliative care health-related interventions in the context of end-of-life, life-threatening, or life-limiting illnesses or conditions. This particular report recognizes but expressly excludes palliative care needs that are not related to the foregoing end-of-life, life threatening, or life-limiting illness or conditions, and that may fall more within the domains of social or spiritual suffering, as well as palliative care interventions that would fall outside of health care.

In this context, the Report (2017, p. 1) identifies a new measure of suffering called "serious health-related suffering," which is associated with illness or injury and physical, emotional, or social suffering and cannot be relieved without medical intervention. In the Report, the Commission also proposes an essential package of palliative care and pain relief services, resources, and interventions that are responsive to "serious health-related suffering" burdens, and recommends social support programs as a complement to this essential package, as delineated below:

- Universal access to an Essential Package by 2030;
- Public financing of The Essential Package for all families at risk of financial catastrophe or impoverishment;
- Basic social supports that complement the Essential Package, financed over and above the health budget in coordination with social welfare programs;
- Policies and additional investment to ensure safe supply chains, to build up human resource capacities through palliative care competency training, and to avoid high costs of pain medications;
- Expanded access to best international pricing for medicines, giving priority to inexpensive, off-patent injectable and oral immediate-release morphine, complemented with necessary technical assistance to ensure safe supply chains and medical use;
- A palliative care and pain relief package for children, taking special account of their specific social and spiritual needs; and
- A UNICEF-led special US$1 million annual fund for children living in low-income countries who are in need of opioids for the relief of pain and palliative care. (See full Panel 16.)

(Knaul et al., 2017, p. 37)

IV. Palliative care and hospice movements in the United States

As part of the evolution of the hospice and palliative care movements in the United States and structures for the delivery and financing of these services, hospice has emerged as a subset of palliative care, and is financed by a separate program benefit known as the Medicare Hospice Benefit. Both movements have made significant contributions to expanding consciousness of an ethic of care among providers, recipients, and caregivers, and in the society at large. At the heart of this transformative philosophy is a therapeutic model that defines the person and the family as the social unit at the center of care, rather than relying solely on the more conventional biomedical model of simply treating disease. As a result of this paradigm shift, in hospice and palliative care the subjective experiences, wishes, values, and preferences of the person and family assume salience in goal setting, advance care planning and decision making. Objective disease and disease treatment become less prominent. Therefore, what is essential to and invariant in the structure of hospice and palliative care is the provision of care to patients, although its intensity may vary. While treatment may cease, care never ceases. A progressive movement in aging and health services is now pushing palliative care out into the community, and contemplating the building of palliative communities and environments that support older adults.

Not surprisingly, with the escalating costs of health care and regional variations in spending and care utilization, there has been much heated debate in health reform over health care programs and benefits, such as Medicare and Medicaid, especially for those who are seriously ill and have advanced life-limiting or life-threatening illness. While there is a structured Medicare Hospice Benefit in the United States, there is no comparable federal benefit for palliative care. The delivery and financing systems for palliative care continue to be a patchwork quilt of programs and benefits. Ironically, in the policy debates that raged fiercely in the period leading up to the federal health reform legislation in 2010 (Patient Protection and Affordable Care Act, 2010), concerns about access to and adequacy of care for the uninsured or underinsured, health disparities, or values of adequacy, equity, and health care justice (Sulmasy, 2003), were subsidiary to concerns about limits on resource use for those who already have health benefits, such as people who are covered by employment-based health insurance or are Medicare program beneficiaries. Most Americans have been reluctant to accept any limits on resource use, or any form of rationing that might be seen as an infringement upon their liberty interest. Except for public discourse about explicit and implicit forms of rationing in which Daniel Callahan (2011) has dared to engage us, myths persist among a broad swath of Americans who continue to believe that higher spending and unlimited resource use mean better quality of care. Adopting an explicit public health perspective, we acknowledge the important and significant role of education and its associated determinants of health in shaping health outcomes, as supported by research evidence (Bossuyt et al., 2011; Olshansky et al., 2012).

How are palliative care and hospice changing this picture? First, we now know that both have the potential to be highly successful health care delivery systems as evidence continues to mount that they are effective models in saving costs (Morrison et al., 2011). They are also associated with good outcomes for patients and families in serious illness and at the end of life, such as controlling pain and symptoms, optimizing quality of life, providing comfort care including comfort feeding, and in some instances extending survival (Mitchell et al., 2009; Palacek et al., 2010; Temel at al., 2010). Hospice utilization has increased dramatically, and in some health care sectors at such a rate that it has drawn the attention of federal regulators (Office of Inspector General, 2016), who continue to demonstrate a somewhat limited understanding of the complexity of the needs of the non-cancer, terminally ill population served by hospice. Drawing from the 2017 report of the Medicare Payment

Advisory Commission (MedPAC), nearly 1.4 million Medicare beneficiaries used hospice services in 2015, a 4.3% increase from 2014. Of the total 2015 Medicare beneficiary decedents, 48.6% used hospice, an increase from 47.9% in 2014. Between 2014 and 2015, there was a slight decline in average length of stay among decedents, from 88.2 days to 86.7 days. This reflects an especially pronounced decrease among those patients with the longest stays. The 2015 median length of stay for hospice decedents was 17 days, a figure that has remained stable at approximately 17 or 18 days for more than a decade (MedPAC, 2017). According to this MedPAC Report, there was continued variation in hospice use in 2017 by demographic and beneficiary characteristics. Medicare decedents who were older, white, female, Medicare Advantage enrollees, living in urban areas or not dual-eligible were more likely to use hospice than their respective counterparts. The most recent *Palliative Care Report Card* from the Center to Advance Palliative Care and the National Palliative Care Research Center indicates that 67% of U.S. hospitals have palliative care teams, and approximately one-third do not (Center to Advance Palliative Care, 2015; Dumanovsky, et al., 2015).

Yet, concerns persist about the goals of palliative care and hospice, and the grounds for withholding and withdrawing life-sustaining treatments for seriously ill individuals who may be subjected to prolonged pain and suffering as the result of medically unnecessary and avoidable interventions. Such decisions to forgo life-sustaining treatments are often associated with hospice and palliative care and may attach certain stigma to utilization of these programs, although the evaluation of end-of-life options also takes place at the hospital bedside, in nursing homes, and assisted living residences that may have no hospice or palliative care programs, and as part of appropriate advance care planning sometimes well before the onset of illness. However, the palliative approach places a prominent emphasis on communication, goals of care discussions, and the decision process that involves valuing one's care choices. Persons who are living through suffering or illness burden, or anticipate such lived experiences, go through a process of attaching value attributes to their suffering experiences in which the emotions play a strong role (Morrissey, 2011a). Suffering persons may value life-prolonging treatments negatively based upon their emotional responses and states, as they discern that these treatments will heighten their suffering burden without providing any benefit such as improving function or quality of life.

There are important distinctions to be made between care that is beneficial, non-beneficial, or only marginally beneficial (Jennings & Morrissey, 2011). While decisions about beneficial and non-beneficial care may engender less disagreement, it is in the marginally beneficial category where there may be reasonable disagreement not only about outcomes for patients, but about their suffering and illness burden and how they would value such experiences (Jennings & Morrissey, 2011). These distinctions are made in the context of a decision process that is implemented in care settings that vary, and in some instances are more restrictive than others. Although it is impossible to provide an exhaustive review of such variations in this chapter, the following brief descriptions of therapeutic care models and settings are provided to help clarify what older persons may face when navigating care transitions and negotiating the evaluation and decision process in serious illness.

A. Palliative care

Palliative care is a therapeutic model and delivery system that can provide both disease-modifying therapy and varying levels of care to the patient, depending upon the patient's medical needs and goals of care. It can be provided as part of hospice or outside of hospice, that is, non-hospice palliative care. "Upstream palliative care" is the term used to describe care that targets chronically ill individuals in earlier stages of illness. Typically, as a patient's serious illness progresses, the balance shifts from principally curative to more intensive levels of palliative and comfort care (Fins, 2006). Palliative care can be accessed in the hospital, nursing home, or community, and generally aims to strengthen communication among patients, family members, surrogates and health professionals, improve care coordination, enhance quality of life, and relieve pain and suffering. The National Consensus Project for Quality Palliative Care (NCP) (2013), citing the U.S. Department of Health and Human Services, the Centers for Medicare & Medicaid Services, and the National Quality Forum, defines palliative care in the following way:

> Palliative care means patient and family-centered care that optimizes quality of life by anticipating, preventing, and treating suffering. Palliative care throughout the continuum of the illness involves addressing physical, intellectual, emotional, spiritual and social needs, and to facilitate patient autonomy, access to information, and choice.
>
> (p. 9)

The NCP (2013) identifies and addresses eight domains of care: (1) structure and processes; (2) physical aspects; (3) psychological and psychiatric aspects; (4) social aspects, (5) spiritual, religious and existential aspects, (6) cultural aspects, (7) care of the patient at end of life, and (8) ethical and legal aspects. (National Consensus Project, 2013, pp. 10–11)

B. Hospice care

Hospice care is a comprehensive interdisciplinary program that provides pain and symptom management as well as psychosocial, emotional, and spiritual support services to patients. While there is sometimes confusion about the relationship between hospice and palliative care, the former is one form or subset of palliative care (Jennings, Ryndes, D'Onofrio, & Baily, 2003) that serves patients who have been certified by their physician to have a life expectancy of six months or less. This eligibility criterion is a requirement of the Medicare Hospice Benefit (MHB), the primary financing mechanism for hospice care. As a result of the MHB, access to hospice care is more restrictive than palliative care. Regular Medicare coverage is suspended for patients who are on the MHB, and providers are reimbursed only for services that are primarily palliative and have a palliative intent. Admission to hospice usually also requires the patient's understanding and agreement to forgo curative medical treatment, although as an exception to the general rule some hospices have "open access" policies that permit curative treatment at the same time as comfort care. Many hospice patients have Do Not Resuscitate (DNR) Orders, which is an order to forgo cardiopulmonary resuscitation (CPR)—a life-sustaining treatment—when there is no pulse or breathing.

C.   Hospital-based care

Hospital-based care is increasingly providing access to both palliative care programs and hospice. Program models may vary from hospital to hospital. Patients or their surrogates will evaluate their palliative and end-of-life options as part of the decision-making process in the hospital. Transfers to acute settings may add additional complexity to the evaluation and decision-making process, especially as such transfers typically involve curative approaches to care and evaluation of more aggressive treatment options.

D.   Nursing home care

Nursing facilities also provide hospice, and in many instances integrate palliative care into the institution's standards of care. Non-hospice nursing home residents or their surrogates also evaluate their palliative and end-of-life options as part of making medical decisions. Decisions involving the withholding or withdrawal of life-sustaining treatment in nursing homes may be subject to additional restrictions, such as ethics committee review.

E.   Community-based care

Hospice care is provided to patients in the community. Innovative models of palliative care are also being embedded in the community. Patients in the community must go through the same decision and valuing process as patients in hospitals and nursing homes and weigh their palliative and end-of-life options. DNR Orders, and sometimes Do Not Intubate (DNI) Orders, are typically available in the community, although surrogates may be subject to restrictions when it comes to other types of life-sustaining treatment decisions.

It is clear from the above descriptions that making decisions about care for older persons is a process that may be potentially fraught with risk, especially risk for confusion about care options and care settings. And it is not only older persons who may be at risk of becoming confused, but aging and health professionals themselves and those who are supporting them. The structural complexity characterizing the aging and health care systems and health care decision making—in particular decision making about palliative and end-of-life options—requires comprehensive education for professionals, older adults, and their caregivers. In most cases, education lags behind the implementation curve of new laws and regulations. This complexity and lack of knowledge create fertile ground for conflict when a loved one is sick. Such conflict frequently occurs within the family, and if it cannot be resolved through informal processes or ethics committee review, it may escalate and end up in the courts. This is an undesirable outcome for everyone involved. How may physicians and health professionals exercise their professional ethical responsibilities when family members are making demands for treatments that are often non-beneficial or marginally beneficial, and could be described as "futile?" How can cases that are conflict-laden be kept out of the courts?

VII.   Futile treatment: How is it defined?

The term "futility" has more than one meaning when used to describe medical treatment. In its original formulation, futile treatment means an intervention that is not effective or would not be successful. The treatment evaluation is based upon physiological evidence of treatment failure or ineffectiveness. According to Joseph J. Fins (2006), futility can be understood both quantitatively and qualitatively. Using the narrowest physiologic basis, a determination of futility is tied to failure in the last 100 cases, although application of this measure in the clinical setting poses challenges (Fins, 2006). Fins explains that futile literally means leaky. For example, in the event of a cardiac arrest, CPR is futile if the resuscitation is not successful and efforts to resuscitate have to be halted.

However, futility has taken on a broader meaning of having no benefit for the patient in ways that go beyond physiological evidence, that is, failing to improve quality of life or function, or failing to relieve pain and suffering. It is in the penumbras of this multidimensional meaning of futility that there has been a much greater difficulty navigating decision about when treatment should cease. Fins (2006) correctly points out that most futility disputes about what constitutes medically and ethically appropriate care arise from communication breakdowns among the patient, family and physician.

Thus far, the principles, policies and decision-making considerations entailed in the "palliative turn" have been couched in largely general terms, as part of a more conceptual discussion. But what does this look like up close? How might the kind of conflicts and communication breakdowns that so often arise in the palliative context play out in specific instances, at ground level? In a book such as this one, which is premised on the intimate relationship of theory with practice and the urgency of engaging with aging Americans as real, flesh-and-blood individuals, it is all the more crucial that we be able to give a face and name to what we are speaking of. With this in mind, we will now turn to a concrete case study that situates some of these dilemmas in a real-life context.

VIII. Case Study: Nursing home resident with dementia

A court decision in New York is illustrative of the complexity of decision making at the end of life, the role of family conflict and the opportunity for palliative care interventions. The case of *Matter of Zornow* (2010) involved a 93-year-old woman, Mrs. Zornow, who resided in a nursing home and had advanced Alzheimer's disease. This is not an uncommon situation in the United States. The majority of nursing home residents are chronically ill, frail elderly women, many of who will at some point in their illness trajectory experience some form of cognitive impairment (Bern-Klug, 2010; Mitchell et al., 2009). In a multi-site study of nursing home residents with advanced dementia conducted by Mitchell and colleagues (2009) in Boston, over 85% of the study participants were women, and Alzheimer's disease was found to be the most prevalent type of dementia.

Mrs. Zornow had a number of things in her favor as she approached the end of life that might have prevented adverse outcomes. First and foremost, she was blessed with seven children. In addition, she had a DNR Order in place. Mrs. Zornow also had two medical orders for life-sustaining treatment (MOLST) Orders, signed by a physician that documented her wishes to forgo artificial nutrition and hydration.

However, as is also not uncommon, a conflict arose between a daughter and the six other children about Mrs. Zornow's wishes. In a petition to the court for the appointment of a guardian, the court made a number of findings, revoked the MOLST Orders, and appointed co-guardians to make decisions for Mrs. Zornow based upon Catholic teaching (*Matter of Zornow*, 2010). This case was decided under New York's family decision making law called the Family Health Care Decisions Act (FHCDA), effective June 2010 (New York Public Health Law [PHL] Art. 29-CC), that authorized public health law surrogates to make decisions for incapable patients who have neither appointed a health care agent nor have any prior directives.

Below is a summary of the 2010 court findings and the order as reported by Mental Hygiene Legal Services:

> A guardian of the person was appointed to make major medical and end-of-life medical decisions as the statutory surrogate under the Family Health Care Decisions Act (FHCDA) for a ward who was a devout Catholic. Under FHCDA the guardian was obliged to make that decision in accordance with the ward's religious beliefs. The Court observed the irony that with respect to artificial hydration and nutrition, had there been a health care proxy (HCP) executed in favor of a most trusted friend or relative, the statutory presumption would have been in favor of artificial

hydration and nutrition, but absent the HCP, under the FHCDA, the presumption is against it because the "quality of life" ethic is paramount under the FHCDA rather than the "sanctity of life" ethic. The court discusses Catholic doctrine in great detail, and concludes that under the "sanctity of life" doctrine of the Church, in nearly every instance, hydration and nutrition, even when administered artificially, are considered by the Church to be "ordinary" rather than "extraordinary" measures, and that hydration and nutrition must be administered except under certain very rare and narrow exceptions which are also discussed in great detail. The court also holds that with respect to end-of-life decisions, the guardians should consult with and obtain the advice of a priest or someone well trained in Catholic moral theology, as is recommended for in the Catholic Guide to End-of-Life Decisions by the National Catholic Bioethics Center.

(Mental Hygiene Legal Service, Second Judicial Department, 2011, p. 98)

As this summary suggests, everything that could have gone wrong certainly went awry with this case, including the court decision itself, which departs wildly from any reasoned understanding of the law. It is also of note that a very lengthy discussion of Catholic dogma in the full decision manages to significantly muddy the waters as to the key issues for Mrs. Zornow's goals of care. This focus on the teachings of a particular faith draws attention away from the central issues in the case concerning goals of care, and medically and ethically appropriate care in light of those goals, which we discuss more fully below.

A.   Discussion and analysis

In light of the complex medical, social, legal and ethical issues involved in the case selected for discussion, we identify the following ten questions that are helpful in analyzing the case and guiding the discussion:

- Who is the older person, what are the older person's known social and medical history, and what are the current clinical diagnoses?
- Does the older person have capacity? If not, are there prior directives? Is there an identified surrogate decision maker?
- What are the proposed alternative treatments that are at issue?
- What are the goals of care?
- Does treatment offer any promise for recovery?
- What is the evaluation of the resident's suffering and illness burden?
- What values enter into the evaluation of benefits and burdens, and appropriate care?
- Is life-sustaining treatment medically and ethically appropriate?
- What informal processes are available in the clinical setting to resolve conflict?
- What is the role of the institutional ethics committee?

B. Description of older person, older person's history and diagnosis

Based upon what is known from two court decisions, Mrs. Zornow was of advancing age at 93 years old, and had advanced Alzheimer's disease (*Matter of Zornow*, 2010). She had been residing in a nursing home in New York State. The court described the irreversible nature of her condition, and with the progression of the disease the risks of developing swallowing difficulties and secondary infections that might lead to death. Advanced dementia is generally viewed and accepted as an irreversible and incurable illness, among the leading causes of death in the United States (Palacek et al., 2010). Mitchell and colleagues (2009) describe patients with advanced dementia as end-stage, not always appropriately recognized as such, and consequently also at risk for receiving less than optimal palliative care. Therefore, based upon this evidence, we may comfortably conclude that Mrs. Zornow was approaching the end of her life, although she may not have met the definition of terminal illness for the purposes of the Medicare Hospice Benefit or other statutory criteria.

In her early illness and prior to being admitted to the nursing home, we learn from the court record that Mrs. Zornow was taken care of by her daughter, Carole Zornow, who had petitioned the court to be her guardian. There were six other siblings who had been involved in their mother's care issues. The court appointed Carole Zornow and her brother, Douglas, as temporary co-guardians in July 2010. The final order of the court appointed Carole Zornow and a Catholic agency as co-guardians for Mrs. Zornow.

C. Capacity, prior directives, and surrogacy

We can infer from the court decision that at the time this matter came before the court in May 2010, Mrs. Zornow probably did not have capacity to make decisions (*Matter of Zornow*, 2010). She had never appointed a health care agent under New York State Law. However, under the New York family decision making statute that became effective in June 2010, a guardian is a legally authorized surrogate under the law. The guardians appointed by the court for Mrs. Zornow acted as public health law surrogates under this statute.

With respect to prior directives, Mrs. Zornow had a DNR Order, and two MOLST Orders, executed successively on September 15 and September 18, 2009 (*Matter of Zornow*, 2010). It is not entirely clear from the court decision whether Mrs. Zornow consented to the MOLST Orders herself while she still had capacity or whether "clear and convincing evidence" was used to complete the MOLST forms, which is permissible under New York State law.

The judge in the case, however, appeared unfamiliar with MOLST Orders and their legal basis in state law. A MOLST Order is consented to by the patient or resident (or if the patient does not have capacity by the surrogate) and signed by a physician and documents the patient's wishes about future care. It is modeled on the national POLST Paradigm, or Physician Orders for Life-Sustaining Treatment. The New York Public Health law was amended in 2008 to permit alternative DNR forms. The MOLST form is an approved New York State Department of Health form that can be used to document DNR, DNI, and Do Not Hospitalize Orders, as well as election of certain levels of care (full treatment, limited interventions, comfort care). The MOLST/POLST paradigm is also supported by a strong evidence base that demonstrates its effectiveness in assuring that patient wishes are honored (Hickman et al., 2009, 2010). Charles Sabatino of the American Bar Association and Naomi Karp of AARP (Sabatino & Karp, 2011) collaborated in the writing of a comprehensive report about POLST that describes its history, how it differs from traditional advance directives, state-by-state developments, and community partnerships that have been instrumental in growing support for the paradigm.

The two MOLST Orders for Mrs. Zornow contained orders not to initiate administration of artificial nutrition and hydration, and not to transfer Mrs. Zornow to the hospital unless she had pain or symptoms that could not be controlled in the nursing home (*Matter of Zornow*, 2010). MOLST Orders are appropriate for seriously, chronically ill individuals who may have less than a year to live. Therefore, this was an appropriate planning tool for Mrs. Zornow. Had Mrs. Zornow not been able to consent to the MOLST Orders herself due to lack of capacity, in the absence of a surrogate, clear and convincing evidence of her wishes could have been used as a basis for completing the MOLST Orders. Her son, Donald, presented evidence at some point that his mother had given verbal instructions to him and his other siblings that she did not want life-sustaining artificial nutrition and hydration if she was no longer able to take in food or water orally.

D.   Proposed alternative treatments

The issue in this case centers on artificial nutrition and hydration, which is a medical treatment under applicable New York statutes. The court revoked Mrs. Zornow's prior MOLST Orders and limitations on treatment. The surrogate therefore was faced with evaluating two options under the life-sustaining treatment standards of the applicable state statute: life-sustaining artificial nutrition and hydration, or forgoing life-sustaining artificial nutrition and hydration and Mrs. Zornow's dying a natural death.

For a patient who is neither terminally ill nor unconscious and has an irreversible or incurable condition, as was the case for Mrs. Zornow, the standards under which the surrogate would have had to evaluate these two options are the following, "Treatment would involve such pain, suffering or other burden that it would reasonably be deemed inhumane or extraordinarily burdensome under the circumstances *and* patient has an irreversible or incurable condition, as determined by attending physician with concurrence" (New York Public Health Law Art. 29-CC).

It should be noted that this standard does not contain any language that explicitly addresses futility. In New York, the Family Health Care Decisions Act eliminated the express futility language that was in the old New York DNR law (New York Public Health Law Art 29-B) that was based upon a physiologic evaluation of futility. However, this change does not bar consideration of futility under the standards. The standards are written more broadly to take in account physiologic bases for futility, as well as qualitative assessment of suffering and illness burden (Morrissey, 2011b). Decisions not relating to CPR that fall under this standard for residents in a nursing home also must be reviewed by the institutional ethics review committee (New York Public Health Law Art. 29-CC).

E.   *Goals of care, promise for recovery, and evaluation of suffering burden*

Mrs. Zornow's case called for evaluation of her suffering burden under the applicable standards. What would that evaluation have involved? In order to properly evaluate suffering burden, it is important to know the older person's goals of care. This is a dialogue that continues over time, because goals of care change as the patient's or resident's clinical course changes. In light of Mrs. Zornow's advanced dementia and irreversible and incurable illness trajectory, the goals of care that would have been discussed with the patient's family or surrogate decision maker fall into three domains: prolonging life; improving quality of life and/or functional status; or enabling potential curative therapy or reversing the disease (PEGS Workgroup, 2017). Decisions about artificial nutrition and hydration, especially tube feeding, tend to create tension and conflict for patients, families and surrogate decision makers because of the emotional responses involved in making such decisions. Family members may discern benefits in tube feeding to the extent such treatment allows them to spend more time with their loved ones and may help to relieve them of feelings of guilt about forgoing treatment options. According to Palacek and colleagues (2010), discussions about feeding tubes also raise a specter for the family of choosing between care or no-care options for the family's loved one, a dichotomy which is not well-founded and the source of serious misconceptions about hospice and palliative care.

In light of Mrs. Zornow's clinical health status, it would have been unlikely she would have experienced any proposed treatment benefits in any of the three domains. The questions that would have had to be asked and carefully weighed about Mrs. Zornow's care would have been:

- Will treatment make a difference?
- Do burdens of treatment outweigh benefits?
- Is there hope of recovery?
- What does the older person value? (Bomba, Morrissey, & Leven, 2011)

In considering these questions with respect to the proposed artificial and nutrition treatment for Mrs. Zornow, her clinical as well as psychosocial and emotional health status would have had to be assessed. Evaluation of pain and suffering require a multidimensional assessment (Altilio, 2004; Morrissey, 2011a). In conducting such a comprehensive assessment, it would be necessary to determine whether the burdens that artificial nutrition and hydration would have imposed on Mrs. Zornow's already compromised systems would have been outweighed by the benefits.

There is strong evidence that frail elderly residents in nursing homes are at high risk for feeding tubes, and that feeding tube interventions are a medical treatment that is associated with poor outcomes for frail elderly persons (Finucane et al., 1999; Mitchell, 2007; Mitchell et al., 2009; Teno et al., 2010). Finucane and colleagues (1999) provide clinical evidence that feeding tubes in patients with dementia do not improve survival and can increase risk of aspiration pneumonia, infections and pressure sores while providing no clear benefits in terms of improving function or providing comfort (Finucane et al., 1999). These complications can heighten the resident's pain and suffering. Based upon the clinical evidence, feeding tubes would likely not have made a difference in Mrs. Zornow's illness course in terms of recovery, and might actually have shortened her survival time.

The alternative for Mrs. Zornow would have been oral or careful hand feeding (Palacek et al., 2010). The benefits of oral feeding would have been enjoyment of the taste and texture of the food, even if what would have been offered were ice chips or ice cream, and the additional benefits of social interaction that oral feeding would have had. Research has also demonstrated that family members find relief in participating in "comfort feeding" (Palacek et al., 2010).

The goals of care discussion for an elderly nursing home resident such as Mrs. Zornow should focus among other things on what she would value, including her known spiritual and religious beliefs. Prior directives, even if not legally valid as stand-alone documents, may be used as evidence of an older person's wishes and values by the surrogate decision maker. In light of Mrs. Zornow's clinical course as an advanced dementia patient and no promise of recovery, as well as the values her prior directives reflected not to be subjected to prolonged suffering, discussion about goals of care would have focused largely on palliation and comfort care—maintaining Mrs. Zornow's quality of life to the extent possible, reducing pain levels, and preventing and relieving suffering. Aggressive treatments such as surgery, dialysis, chemotherapy, or feeding tubes would in most cases be medically inappropriate for an advanced dementia patient. Mrs. Zornow would have been an appropriate candidate for palliative care or hospice care.

F.   Social history and social and cultural contexts

The Mrs. Zornow case is not an uncommon scenario, although usually conflicts such as the ones that arose in this case are resolved informally or at the ethics committee level before they reach the courts. The courts should continue to be viewed as arbiters of last resort. The Zornow case demonstrates how important social history, and social and cultural contexts, are to end-of-life decision making. Appropriate social, emotional and spiritual supports in dealing with the struggles older persons face are core constituents of good end-of-life care.

G. Health care justice

What steps should be taken when health professionals are faced with requests for medical treatment that clearly exceed standards of reasonableness in light of a seriously ill older person's goals of care, or when no conventional medical treatments or interventions seem to make sense, either medically or ethically? Benefits-burdens analysis and evaluation of the older person's suffering are essential tools in clinical ethics. Questions concerning health care justice and equitable allocation of scarce resources also come into play. Evaluation of provision of non-beneficial or marginally beneficial, and oftentimes harmful, interventions to older persons with serious illness such as advanced dementia, may call for appropriate ethics consultation (Jennings & Morrissey, 2011). Information about palliative and end-of-life care options should be provided to the older person or her/his health care agent or surrogate decision maker.

IX. Recommendations: The four-pronged approach of the public health strategy for palliative care

Consistent with the public health strategy for palliative care, we call for a four-pronged approach to help address the problem of unreasonable and unjust demand and unmet palliative care needs: (1) national policy making; (2) assuring access to essential medicines; (3) education and training for aging and health professionals, including judges and community workers, about palliative care; and (4) policy implementation, including at the systems level.

A. National-level policy

A call for federal legislation on palliative care aligns with the first key component of the public health strategy—namely, development of national policy. Enactment of federal legislation that would create a federal right to palliative care in the United States and provide funding for such programs is a priority, as called for by the Lancet Commission (Knaul et al., 2017). U.S. federal agencies have begun to take incremental steps to address the public health problem of pain, an important focus of palliative care.

National-level policy on palliative care may also be influenced by professional associations and advocacy organizations that have adopted their own policies or resolutions on palliative care, such as the American Public Health Association (Morrissey & Miller, 2013), the American Heart Association (Braun et al., 2016), and the American Psychological Association (2017).

B.   *Availability of essential medicines*

Federal- and state-level policy must assure the availability of essential medicines, such as opioids. On October 26, 2017, the President of the United States declared the opioid crisis in the United States a national public health emergency under federal law. Even in light of the declaration of this national public health emergency, persons with serious illness and chronic pain or intolerable and intractable pain still have a right to access the full range of medicines they need to relieve and control their pain. The *Lancet* Commission Report, "Alleviating the access abyss in palliative care and pain relief—an imperative of universal coverage" (Knaul et al., 2017), recognizes the need for balance in assuring both the safe use of opioids, and reducing the risks of diversion and conflicts of interest:

> The crisis in the USA provides lessons on the need for maximising the benefits of opioids and minimising the risk of non-medical use as access to opioid analgesics is increased in a step-wise manner in LMICs. Countries should monitor the supply and marketing of opioids and implement strong conflict-of-interest policies to restrict undue influence of all for-profit entities in the tendering, procurement, and marketing of opioid medications and in describing indications for use and prescription of opioid medications. These policies must also guarantee training on safe use of opioid analgesics grounded in evidence-based protocols.
>
> (Knaul et al., 2017, p. 12)

The 2011 report by the Institute of Medicine (IOM), *Relieving Pain in America*, drew attention to the seriousness and magnitude of the public health problem of pain and the over 100 million adults living with chronic pain. In response to the IOM's recommendation, the Department of Health & Human Services created the Interagency Pain Research Coordinating Committee that coordinated the development of a "National Pain Strategy, A Comprehensive Population Health-Level Strategy for Pain" (NPS) (2016). The NPS addresses six key areas: population research, prevention and care, disparities, service delivery and payment, professional education and training, and public education and communication.

In addition, the National Institutes of Health Office of Pain Policy has released its Federal Pain Research Strategy (FPRS) (2017), an effort that was also overseen by the Interagency Pain Research Coordinating Committee. The FPRS is directed to all federal agencies and departments that are involved in pain research.

C.   Education

There is a widespread consensus that we need to lay much stronger foundations in palliative and end-of-life care when it comes to the education and training we provide to our aging and health professionals and para-professionals, in multiple domains including pain management, ethics, and ethical dilemmas. Content that focuses only on new laws and regulations is not sufficient. The really important education must target the translation of mandates on palliative care and pain relief into meaningful person-centered care on the ground for all persons living with serious illness or chronic pain, including older persons, their families and health professionals who are situated in different health care settings, especially as these seriously ill older adults make care transitions from one setting to another. Funding for education and training is desperately needed and will go a long way to address deficits in knowledge about geriatric health and palliative systems of care, as well as applicable laws and regulations and their implications, which may be contributing to bad outcomes for patients and families. Federal workforce grants have been one source of funding for such education. (See Appendix F, Finger Lakes Geriatric Education Center—Geriatrics Workforce Enhancement Program.)

D.   *Policy implementation and systems-level change*

Hospice is a model of care that effectuates change at the systems level. It is both a philosophy of care and a delivery system. Patients who consent to hospice care are informed that they are forgoing primarily curative care when they transition into hospice. Decisions made at the systems level, such as in the hospice model, relieve crisis and conflict at the bedside. Robert Burt (2005) advances three "countervailing schemes" to alter decision making processes:

1   No one should be socially authorized to engage in conduct that directly, purposefully, and unambiguously inflicts death, whether on another person or on oneself.
2   Decisions that indirectly lead to death should be acted upon only after a consensus is reached among many people. No single individual should be socially authorized to exercise exclusive control over decisions that might lead to death, whether that individual is the dying person, the attending physician, or a family member acting as health care proxy.
3   As much as possible, end-of-life care should not depend on explicit decisions made at the bedside of a specific dying person, but rather should be implicitly dictated by systems-wide decisions about available resources, personnel, and institutional settings—that is, by setting up default pathways that implicitly guide and even control caretaking decisions in individual cases.

(Burt, 2005, p. S11)

Burt's proposed end-of-life decision making scheme would support the paradigm shift that is already occurring in palliative and end-of-life care toward more communitarian, social and relational models. Such models recognize autonomy, but in the larger social ecological context of community.

Hospitals and nursing homes can begin to make systems decisions that are modeled on hospice care, such as what level of resources to allocate to ICU units, perhaps limiting access to days spent in the ICU, or integrating palliative care into standards of care, thus making palliative care accessible to all residents. As Burt suggests, changes at the systems level will help to mitigate conflict-laden and emotionally stressful end-of-life choices for families and surrogates at the very time when they need to be investing their emotional resources in relational time and communication with their loved ones.

1.   Improved care coordination, communication, and interdisciplinary team care planning processes

Consistent with the POLST/MOLST evidence-based paradigm and process for documenting goals of care discussions, the decision process about artificial nutrition and hydration and levels of care such as those at issue in *Matter of Zornow*, as well as other forms of life-sustaining treatment, should begin with early conversations with social workers and other members of the interdisciplinary team who can explain care options to families and surrogates, including the option to provide "comfort only" feeding to patients for whom tube feeding is not medically or ethically appropriate (Palacek et al., 2010). Goals of care and preference-sensitive treatment decisions can be translated into medical orders and reviewed periodically by the patient's physician and other health care professionals. One of the strengths of social work involvement in the POLST/MOLST program is the opportunity to improve communication and care coordination among patients, physicians, family members, caregivers, health care agents, or surrogates. Communication has been identified as critically important to person-centered care, shared decision-making process and preference-concordant care, and instrumental in avoiding futility disputes (Bomba, Morrissey, & Leven, 2011; Fins, 2006).

2.   Ethics consultation and ethics committee review

In many states, statutes mandate that certain cases be reviewed by institutional ethics review committees. For example, New York law requires that all life-sustaining treatment decisions for nursing home residents who are neither terminally ill nor permanently unconscious (except for decisions about CPR) be reviewed by the ethics committee. The decision of the ethics committee in these cases is binding. Even for non-mandated reviews, physicians or anyone connected with a case may refer a case to the ethics committee for advice or in the event of a conflict such as between a physician and a patient, or between surrogates. Many facilities that have the necessary trained and qualified staff will make ethics consultations available without convening the full committee. Ethics consultations and ethics committees should be seen as essential resources for patients, families, and health professionals to help resolve disputes where conflict may seem intractable. Ethics committee members must also receive appropriate training instructing them in the serious responsibilities they assume in serving in this role (Morrissey, 2011b). In the case referenced in this chapter, *Matter of Zornow*, contested decisions about appropriate care for seriously ill older persons who may not be terminally ill would have been reviewed by the respective institutional ethics committee, under the mandates of the applicable state statute. Assuring that ethics committee members have immunity from liability for their good-faith participation in the ethics committee process is also a *sine qua non* of policy making in this area.

X.   Conclusion

A public health strategy for palliative care holds great promise for strengthening older persons' equitable access to palliative systems of care that aim to relieve suffering and improve quality of life. The key components of that strategy—policy development, drug availability, education, and policy implementation—provide a blueprint for progressive change in elder care. Pushing the boundaries of palliative care into the community and embedding the palliative approach in home- and community-based services will be the most effective in translating policy into meaningful interventions for frail and seriously ill older persons, and avoiding unjust demands for futile, non-beneficial or marginally beneficial treatments by family members or surrogates.

Acknowledgment

Mary Beth Quaranta Morrissey acknowledges first publication of parts of this chapter by Hospice Foundation of America in Chapter 12, "Unjust Demands for Treatment: When Treatment Should Cease," in K.J. Doka, A.S. Tucci, C.A. Corr, & B. Jennings (Eds.). (2012). *End-of-Life Ethics: A Case Study Approach*. Washington, DC: Hospice Foundation of America.

References

Altilio, T. (2004). Pain and symptom management: An essential role for social work. In J. Berzoff & P.R. Silverman (Eds.), *Living with dying: Handbook for end-of-life healthcare practitioners* (pp. 380–408). New York: Columbia University Press.
American Psychological Association. (2017). Resolution on palliative care and end-of-life issues. Retrieved from: www.apa.org/about/policy/palliative-care-eol.aspx
Bern-Klug, M. (2010). Trends in the characteristics of nursing homes and residents. In M. Bern-Klug (Ed.), *Transforming palliative care in nursing homes* (pp. 84–106). New York: Columbia University Press.

Bomba, P., Morrissey, M.B., & Leven, D.C. (2011). Key role of social work in effective communication and conflict resolution process: Medical orders for life-sustaining treatment (MOLST) program in New York and shared medical decision making at the end of life. *Journal of Social Work in End-of-Life and Palliative Care, 7*(1), 56–82.

Bossuyt, N., Van den Block, L., Cohen, J., Meeussen, K., Bilsen, J., Echteld M., ... Van Casteren, V. (2011). Is individual educational level related to end-of-life care use? Results from a nationwide retrospective cohort study in Belgium. *Journal of Palliative Medicine, 14*(10), 1135–1141.

Braun, L.T., Grady, K.L., Kutner, J.S., Adler, E., Berlinger, N., Boss, R., ... Roach, W.H., and on behalf of the American Heart Association Advocacy Coordinating Committee. (2016). Palliative care and cardiovascular disease and stroke. A policy statement from the American Heart Association and American Stroke Association. *Circulation, 134*(11). https://doi.org/10.1161/CIR.0000000000000438

Burt, R. (2005). The end of autonomy. *Hastings Center Report Special Supplement, 35*(6), S9–S13.

Callahan, D. (2011). Rationing: Theory, politics, and passions. *Hastings Center Report, 41*(2), 23–27.

Center to Advance Palliative Care (CAPC) (2015). America's care of serious illness: 2015 state-by-state report card on access to palliative care in our nation's hospitals. Retrieved from: https://reportcard.capc.org/

Connor, S., & Sepulveda, C.M. (Eds.) (2014). *Global atlas of palliative care at the end of life*. Geneva/London: World Health Organization and Worldwide Palliative Care Alliance.

Dumanovsky, T., Augustin, R., Rogers, M., Lettang, K., Meier, D.E., & Morrison, R.S. (2015). The growth of palliative care in U.S. hospitals: A status report. *Journal of Palliative Medicine, 19*(1). https://doi.org/10.1089/jpm.2015.0351

Fins, J.J. (2006). *A palliative ethic of care: Clinical wisdom at life's end*. Sudbury, MA: Jones and Bartlett.

Finucane, T.E., Christmas, C., & Travis, K. (1999). Tube feeding in patients with advanced dementia: A review of the evidence. *Journal of the American Medical Association, 282*, 1365–1370.

Gostin, L. (2014). *Global health law*. Cambridge, Mass: Harvard University Press.

Hickman, S.E., Nelson, C.A., Moss, A.H., Hammes, B.J., Terwilliger, A., Jackson, A., & Tolle, W. (2009). Use of the physician orders for life-sustaining treatment (POLST) para digm program in the hospice setting. *Journal of Palliative Medicine, 12*(2), 133–141.

Hickman, S.E., Nelson, C.A., Perrin, N.A., Moss, A.H., Hammes, B.J., & Tolle, S.W. (2010). A comparison of methods to communicate treatment preferences in nursing facilities: Traditional practices versus the physician orders for life-sustaining treatment program. *Journal of American Geriatrics Society, 58*(7), 1241–1248.

Hunt, P. (2007). *Report of the Special Rapporteur on the right of everyone to the highest attainable standard of mental and physical health*. Rep. no. A/HRC/4/28.ECOSOC. Retrieved from: www.ohchr.org/EN/Issues/Health/Pages/SRRightHealthIndex .aspx

Institute of Medicine (IOM). (2011). *Relieving pain in America: A blueprint for transforming prevention, care, education, and research*. Washington, DC: National Academies Press.

International Association for the Study of Pain (IASP). (2010). Declaration that access to pain management is a fundamental human right. Retrieved from: www .iasp-pain.org/Advocacy/Content.aspx?ItemNumber=1821

Jennings, B., Ryndes, T., D'Onofrio, C., & Baily, M.A. (2003). Access to hospice care: Expanding boundaries, overcoming barriers. *Hasting Center Report Special Supplement*, *33*(2), S3–S7.

Jennings, B.J, & Morrissey, M.B. (2011). Health care costs in end-of-life and palliative care: A quest for ethical reform. *Journal of Social Work in End-of-Life and Palliative Care*, *7*(4), 300–317.

Knaul, F.M., Farmer, P.E., Krakauer, E.L., De Lima, L., Bhadelia, A., Jiang Kwete, X., ... Rajagopal, M.R. (2017). Alleviating the access abyss in palliative care and pain relief—An imperative of universal health coverage: The Lancet Commission Report. *Lancet*. Advance online publication. doi: 10.1016/S0140-6736(17)32513-8

Mann, J., Gostin, L., Bruskin, S., Brennan, T., Lazzarini, Z., & Fineberg, H.V. (1994). Health and human rights. *Health and Human Rights*, *1*, 6–23.

Mather, M., Jacobsen, L.A., & Pollard, K.M. (2015). Aging in the United States. *Population Bulletin*, *70*(2), 1–18.

Matter of Carole Zornow, 31 Misc 3rd 450, 919 N.Y.S.2d 273, (Sup. Ct.,Monroe County, 2010); *Matter of Zornow*, 31 Misc 3d 450; 2010 N.Y. Misc., LEXIS 6589; 2010 NY Slip Op 20549 (Sup. Ct., Monroe Cty. 2010); 34 Misc 3d 1208(A), 2011 NY Misc LEXIS 6441 (NY Sup Ct, Dec. 13, 2011).

Medicare Payment Advisory Commission (MedPAC) (2017, June). *Health care spending and the Medicare program. June 2017 data book.* Washington, DC: Medicare Payment Advisory Commission.

Mental Hygiene Legal Service, Second Judicial Department. (2011). *MHL Article 81 and related matters: Collected cases (current through August 2011).*

Mitchell, S.L. (2007). A 93-year-old man with advanced dementia and eating problems. *Journal of the American Medical Association*, *298*(21), 2527–2536.

Mitchell, S.L., Teno, J.M., Kiely, D.K., Shaffer, M.L., Jones, R.N., Prigerson, H.G., ... Hamel, M.B. (2009). The clinical course of advanced dementia. *New England Journal of Medicine*, *361*(16), 1529–1538.

Morrison, R.S., Dietrich, J., Ladwig, S., Quill, T., Sacco, J., Tangeman, J., & Meier, D.E. (2011). Palliative care consultation teams cut hospital costs for Medicaid beneficiaries. *Health Affairs*, *30*(3), 454–463.

Morrissey, M.B. (2011a). Phenomenology of pain and suffering at the end of life: A humanistic perspective in gerontological health and social work. *Journal of Social Work in End-of-Life and Palliative Care*, *7*(1), 14–38.

Morrissey, M.B. (2011b). Educating ethics review committees in a more humanistic approach to relational decision making. *New York State Bar Association Health Law Journal Special Edition: Implementing the Family Health Care Decisions Act*, *16*(1), 65–67.

Morrissey, M.B., Herr, K., & Levine, C. (2015). Public health imperative of the 21st century: Innovations in palliative care systems, services, and supports to improve health and well-being of older Americans. *Gerontologist*, 1–7. doi:10.1093/geront /gnu178

Morrissey, M.B., & Miller, S. (2013). *American Public Health Association policy statement 2005-9 – Supporting public health's role in addressing unmet needs at the end of life*. Washington, DC: American Public Health Association.

National Consensus Project for Quality Palliative Care. (2013). *Clinical practice guide-lines for quality palliative care, 3rd ed.* Pittsburgh, PA: National Consensus Project for Quality Palliative Care.

National Institutes of Health. (2017). *Federal pain research strategy.* Washington, DC: National Institutes of Health.

National Pain Strategy. (2016). *A comprehensive population health-level strategy for pain.* Washington, DC: U.S. Department of Health & Human Services.

New York Public Health Law Art. 29-CC. Office of Inspector General Department of Health and Human Services. (2011, July). Medicare hospices that focus on nursing facility residents. Washington, DC.

Office of the Inspector General, Department of Health & Human Services. (2016). Hospices inappropriately billed Medicare over $250 million for general inpatient care OEI-02-10-00491. Retrieved from: https://oig.hhs.gov/oei/reports/oei-02-10-00491.pdf

Olshansky, S.J., Antonucci, T., Berkman, L., Binstock, R.H., Boersch-Supan, A., Cacioppo, J.T., … Rowe, J. (2012). Differences in life expectancy due to race and educational differences are widening, and may not catch up. *Health Affairs, 31*(8), 1803–1813.

Palecek, E.J., Teno, J.M., Casarett, D.J., Hanson, L.C., Rhodes, R.L., & Mitchell, S.L. (2010). *Journal of American Geriatrics Society, 58*(3), 580–584.

Patient Protection and Affordable Care Act, 42 U.S.C. § 18001 (2010).

Percutaneous Endoscopic Gastronomy (PEGS) Workgroup. (2017). Community-wide guidelines for long term tube feeding/PEG placement for adults. Retrieved from: www.compassionandsupport.org/index.php/for_professionals/molst_training_center/tube_feeding_peg_s

Sabatino, C., & Karp, N. (2011). *Improving advanced illness care: The evolution of state POLST programs.* Washington, DC: AARP Public Policy Institute.

Sen, A. (2008). Why and how is health a human right? *Lancet, 372,* 2010.

Stjernswärd, J., Foley, K.M., & Ferris, F.D. (2007). The public health strategy for pal-liative care. *Journal of Pain and Symptom Management, 33*(5), 486–493.

Sulmasy, D.P. (2003). Health care justice and hospice care. *Hastings Center Report Special Supplement, 33*(2), S14–S17.

Temel, J.S., Greer, J.A., Muzikansky, A., Gallagher, E.R., Admane, S., Jackson, V.A., … Lynch, T.J. (2010). Early palliative care for patients with metastatic non-small-cell lung cancer. *New England Journal of Medicine, 363,* 733–742.

Teno, J.M., Mitchell, S.L., Gozalo, P.L., Dosa, D., Hsu, A., Intrator, O., & Mor, V. (2010). Hospital characteristics associated with feeding tube placement in nurs-ing home residents with advanced cognitive impairment. *Journal of the American Medical Association, 303*(6), 544–550. doi: 10.1001/jama.2010.79

United Nations. (1948). Universal declaration of human rights, 10 December 1948, 217 A (III). Retrieved from: www.un.org/en/documents/udhr/

United Nations Office of the High Commissioner for Human Rights (OHCHR). (2008). Fact sheet no. 31, The right to health. Retrieved August 13, 2014 from: www.refworld.org/docid/48625a742.html

World Health Organization. (n.d.). WHO definition of palliative care. Retrieved from: www.who.int/cancer/palliative/definition/en

World Health Organization. (2014). *Strengthening of palliative care as a component of comprehensive care throughout the life course. WHA67.19.* Geneva, Switzerland: World Health Organization. Retrieved from: http://apps.who.int/gb/ebwha/pdf_files/WHA67/A67_R19-en.pdf?ua=1&ua=1

World Health Organization. (2016). *Planning and implementing palliative care services: A guide for programme managers.* Geneva, Switzerland: World Health Organization.

Wronka, J. (2008). *Human rights and social justice: Social action and service for the helping and health professions.* Thousand Oaks, CA: SAGE.

Bibliography

American Heart Association/American Stroke Association. (2013, September). Principles for palliative care. Retrieved from: www.heart.org/idc/groups/ahaecc public/@wcm/@adv/documents/downloadable/ucm_467599.pdf

Compassion and Support. (2009). Medical orders for life sustaining treatment—patients and families. Retrieved from: www.compassionandsupport.org/index.php /for_patients_families/molst/patients_family_faqs

Compassion and Support. (2017). Community-wide guidelines for long term tube feeding/PEG placement for adults. Retrieved from: CompassionAndSupport.org

Hunt, P. (2006). *Report of the Special Rapporteur on the right of everyone to the highest attainable standard of mental and physical health.* Rep. no. E/CN.4/2006/48. ECOSOC. Retrieved from: www.ohchr.org/EN/Issues/Health/Pages/SRRightHealthIndex.aspx

Morrison, R.S., & Meier, D. (2015). *America's care of serious illness: A state-by-state report card on access to palliative care in our nation's hospitals.* New York: Center to Advance Palliative Care.

National POLST Paradigm. (2017). Physician orders for life-sustaining treatment program. Retrieved from: www.polst.org/

President's Commission on Combating Drug Addiction and the Opioid Crisis. (2017). Retrieved from: www.whitehouse.gov/sites/whitehouse.gov/files/images/Final_Report _Draft_11-1-2017.pdf

United Nations. (1966). International covenant on economic, social and cultural rights, 16 December 1966, *United Nations, Treaty Series,* 993, 3. Retrieved from: https:// treaties.un.org/Pages/ViewDetails.aspx?mtdsg_no=IV-3&chapter=4&lang=en

United Nations. (2000). Committee on Economic, Social and Cultural Rights (CESCR). General comment no. 14: The right to the highest attainable standard of health (Art. 12 of the Covenant), 11 August 2000, E/C.12/2000/4. Retrieved from: www.un.org/documents/ecosoc/docs/2001/e2001-22.pdf

World Health Organization. (2012). Dementia: A public health priority. Geneva, Switzerland: World Health Organization. Retrieved January 26, 2016 from: www .who.int/mental_health/publications/dementia_report_educatio2012/en/

8 A more humanistic approach to relational decision making

Practical ethics and ethics committees

I. Introduction

An important domain of elder health and well being that is often overlooked in the context of public health is health care decision making. It is a widely held, commonsense belief that health care decisions are made by individuals, and therefore are solely a matter of exercise of individual autonomy and self-determination. However, decisions are always made in social, cultural, and relational contexts and are as much a matter of such contexts as they are about individual choices. A great deal of attention has been given to processes of advance care planning for chronically and seriously ill older adults, particularly in the decades since the enactment of the Patient Self-Determination Act of 1990, state health care proxy and surrogate decision-making laws, and adoption of Physician Orders for Life-Sustaining Treatment (POLST) (or in New York, Medical Orders for Life-Sustaining Treatment [MOLST]) programs by states. While progress has been made through these policy initiatives, the complexity involved in decision making is not always fully accessible through the lens of planning in advance. Decision making merits serious attention and reflection in its own right, especially in light of family conflict that may be encountered by older persons, their agents or surrogates, or health care professionals as part of the process. This chapter examines complexity in processes of decision making, including decision making by surrogates, the utilization of ethics committees as a tool for addressing conflict, and the development of interprofessional education and training curricula for ethics committee members and aging and health care professionals. We use New York law and policy on decision making and palliative care as a case study to illustrate challenges in policy implementation.

It has become increasingly clear to aging and health care professionals and practitioners, as well as policy makers, that there have been unforeseen challenges in implementing laws that govern decision making on the ground in clinical practice settings. We describe this as the domain of practical ethics. Many of these challenges relate to ethical issues and ethical dilemmas in decision making for which there are no prescriptive formulae, such as negotiating sometimes complex relationships and conflicts within families, and between health care professionals and surrogates who may be legally authorized to act for incapable older adults. A more humanistic approach to understanding such relationships and conflicts that draws upon reflective practice strategies and tools may enhance understanding of older persons' and family members' lived experiences of illness burden, pain and suffering, and the fully relational dimensions of the health care decision-making process.

Person-centered care has been hailed as an approach that can drive trans-formations in the health systems. The Affordable Care Act (2010) requires that states receiving federal funds develop person-centered planning standards for home and community-based long-term services. Federal guidance and regula-tions spell out how this approach must be implemented in the health systems. For example, the Centers for Medicare & Medicaid Services (CMS) recently promulgated regulations for long-term care facilities that spell out the require-ments for comprehensive person-centered care planning for each resident, in accordance with resident rights (Centers for Medicare & Medicaid Services, 2016). The Institute of Medicine *Dying in America* report (2015) also calls for delivery of person-centered and family-oriented end-of-life care and recom-mends a palliative approach to such care.

The principles of person-centered care were first developed by psycholo-gist Carl Rogers (1961), who identified unconditional positive regard, congru-ence, and empathic listening as central to interpersonal understanding. This book suggests that these principles should be fully incorporated as part of an "elder-centered care" approach in designing elder systems of care. The goals, values, and preferences of the older person are central to person-, and more specifically, elder-centered care planning processes.

Palliative care is by design a person- and family-centered model of care that aims to improve communication with seriously ill older adults and their caregivers. We call the integration of palliative care into elder care planning and decision making, and across the aging and health systems, the *"palliative turn."*

II.   Case study: New York policy implementation—Health care decision making, surrogacy, ethics committees, and interprofessional education

In this chapter, we use New York State laws on health care decision mak-ing and palliative care as a case study in policy formulation and implementa-tion. New York has passed a number of laws that govern health care decision making, including the NY Health Care Proxy Law (New York Public Health Law Art. 29-C) and NY Family Health Care Decisions Act (New York Public Health Law Art. 29-CC), as well as two palliative care laws—the Palliative Care Information Act (New York Public Health Law Section 2997-c), and the Palliative Care Access Act (New York Public Health Law Section 2997-d). More specifically, we illustrate implementation challenges in surrogate deci-sion making, and describe the case of a nursing home resident who is enrolled in and discharged from hospice. Following this case presentation, we discuss the role of ethics committees and provide a blueprint for an interdisciplinary educational training curricula.

A. Implementation challenges: The example of surrogate decision making

Surrogacy is a process and an outcome that has taken on multiple meanings in palliative and end-of-life care today. Under the U.S. federalist system of government, states have traditionally been the "incubators" of health policy. New York serves as a good example of how such policy developed in the area of health care decision making over the last two decades. In 2010, after 17 years of legislative advocacy, New York was one of the last states to adopt family decision making legislation (New York Public Health Law Art. 29-CC, 2010). Prior to June 2010, there had been no family surrogate in New York State under the public health law—only a health care agent under New York's 1991 Health Care Proxy Law (New York Public Health Law Art. 29-C, 1990) and a type of surrogate decision making under New York's 1987 Do Not Resuscitate Law (New York Public Health Law Art 29-B, 1988), now repealed. For incapable patients who had no health care agent or no prior directive, "clear and convincing" evidence of the patient's wishes was legally required pursuant to the U.S. Supreme Court standard in *Cruzan* (1990). This evidence standard imposed an unreasonable burden on patients, families and health care providers.

All 50 states have some form of surrogacy law and advance directive instruments that permit planning in advance for health care, although the legal requirements differ from state to state. Living wills and health care proxies, known sometimes in other states as durable powers of attorney for health care, have been in effect in most states for a number of years. Advance directives are the product of a rational individualistic paradigm that has prevailed in the United States since the 1980s and resulted in the enactment of the federal Patient Self-Determination Act (1990) and statutes at the state level such as New York's Do Not Resuscitate Law and Health Care Proxy Law. These policy enactments aligned with the social and economic neoliberal policies of the Reagan administration, and the rights-based, contractarian paradigm that is rooted in Western notions of autonomy and self-determination. The values underlying this paradigm are self-interested rational decision making, efficiency, and a free market.

In more recent history, however, this paradigm has been critiqued as being unduly polarizing across class and culture, unreasonably individualistic and rationalistic, and failing to explain pluralistic American values, choices, and behaviors (Meisel, 2003; Morrissey & Jennings, 2006; Sabatino & Karp, 2011). Nationwide only a third of Americans have completed advance directives, with certain pockets of the country achieving higher levels of success, such as Upstate New York. Significant barriers to completion of advance directives have persisted, despite massive efforts to convince the American public that they are an effective tool in assuring that patients' wishes are honored in the health systems. Distrust of the health care system, varying styles of communication, religious values and beliefs, and cultural differences in a diverse society in America have been identified as some of the numerous factors that have undermined the effectiveness of advance directives (Gutheil & Heyman, 2005; Bullock, 2011).

Research evidence has also pointed to outcomes and implementation challenges that run counter to the original policy goals that were formulated to advance autonomy. The SUPPORT (1995) study, conducted at five hospital sites in 1995, examined attitudes toward advance directives and outcomes after an educational intervention by trained health professionals and showed poor communication among patients, families and their physicians, inadequate pain care, little understanding of what patients' advance directives meant and how they could be translated into medical orders in the clinical setting, and continued aggressive interventions at the end of life. Research points to regional variations in use of advance directives, in particular an economic relationship between high-intensity end-of-life care in high-spending regions and increased use of advance directives that limit treatment (Nicholas, Langa, Iwashyna, & Weir, 2011). These trends are consistent with Dartmouth researchers' findings that care, spending, and utilization of health care vary by region and are influenced by local practice patterns and norms (Wennberg, Fisher, Goodman, & Skinner, 2008). Nicholas and colleagues reported that individuals with advance directives were more likely to be white, more highly educated, and wealthy (Nicholas et al., 2011). A study in the ICU of a major oncology center demonstrated that utilization of living wills was higher among individuals who were old or white, and less common among Medicaid beneficiaries (Halpern, Pastores, Chou, Chawla, & Thaler, 2011). Data recently reported by the Kaiser Family Foundation (Dijulio, Hamel, Wu, & Brodie, 2017) are consistent with these studies: those with higher income and more years of education were more likely to have documents describing their medical wishes or appointing a health care proxy. These study findings and data, examined in the context of the Dartmouth research, suggest further inquiry into whether and to what extent advance care planning and end-of-life decision making may be influenced by access to care, social and economic resources, and health literacy. The evidence certainly raises a serious concern about adequate and equitable access to health care, and the presence and prevalence of economic disparities that may be driving health care choices and decisions at the end of life, contributing to broader health disparities among Americans. While the goals of the Patient Self-Determination Act and state-enabling statutes were in part the outgrowth of economic policy, there was at least no explicit goal that advance directives would become an instrument of power and capital.

A new paradigm is taking root in health care that moves away from a purely rights-based view of the legal, transactional formalities of advance directives, toward an ethic of care that focuses on relational processes of communication. This shift toward person-centered care encompasses future-oriented advance care planning that aims to foster process conversations between patients and their physicians. The adoption of a humanistic perspective that is based upon human relationships and development in relation to meaningful others also conceptualizes autonomy and rights as being essentially relational. It is in this relational and social context that surrogates assume and carry out their responsibilities for incapable patients.

The major points of the legal and ethical consensus governing health care decision making that are key to the surrogate decision-making process are the following:

- Competent patients have a constitutional right to refuse medical treatment, including life-sustaining treatment (*Cruzan*, 1990).
- Incompetent patients have a constitutionally protected liberty interest in refusing medical treatment, and their surrogates' decisions may be subject to evidentiary standards (*Cruzan*, 1990).
- Patients have a right to make advance directives (Patient Self-Determination Act, 1990).
- The legal authority of the surrogate generally becomes effective upon the determination of the incapacity of the patient (New York Public Health Law Art. 29-C, Art 29-CC).
- The legal authority of the surrogate generally is limited to decisions about health care treatment (New York Public Health Law Art. 29-C, Art 29-CC).
- Artificial nutrition and hydration is a medical treatment and may be withheld and withdrawn pursuant to a patient's constitutionally protected liberty interest (*Cruzan*, 1990).
- There is no legal and ethical distinction between withholding and withdrawing life-sustaining treatment (Meisel, 2003; Morrissey & Jennings, 2006).
- Active euthanasia and assisted suicide are morally and legally distinct from forgoing life-sustaining treatment (Meisel, 2003; Morrissey & Jennings, 2006, p. 53).

Even in light of this well-established consensus, however, surrogates continue to operate in a radically changing environment as they seek to honor the wishes of their loved ones. The evaluation process in which they are called upon to engage in weighing treatment options is complex and has cognitive, social and emotional dimensions (Morrissey, 2011). The important role of social and emotional support, as well as provision of critical education to surrogates about their responsibilities, is essential to making the decision-making experience for the relational family or social unit a less burdensome and more meaningful one. Here, as in the previous chapter, a case example may be instructive in conveying the full range of dimensions to be considered when evaluating this critically important decision-making process.

B.   Experience of a frail nursing home resident: Care transitions

The following case study is drawn from a research investigation (Morrissey, 2011). However, all information is de-identified. The period described dates from April 2010 through October 2010. During this period, the researcher conducted seven interviews with the study participant.

1.   Medical, social, and family history

M is an 88-year-old black woman residing in a nursing home in a borough of New York City. *M* was admitted to the nursing facility's short-term rehabilitation unit in 2007, and later transferred to the long-term care unit due to her diagnoses and limitations. In the long-term unit, *M* receives 24-hour skilled nursing care.

M was born outside the United States, lost her father at an early age, and was raised by her mother, grandmother, and great-grandmother. She came to the United States, was married twice, but lost both of her husbands to cancer and supported her family on her own. *M* has three children, one of whom is very involved with her care. *M*'s adjustment to the nursing home was somewhat difficult. She is very verbal and makes her needs known to the staff. The staff have made efforts to accommodate her needs and make her feel at home, such as for example, making her tea.

M has both a Health Care Proxy and a Do Not Resuscitate (DNR) Order. *M*'s health care proxy documents the following: "*Do not wish to be on a respirator.*" Her daughter is her health care agent. *M* meets clinical criteria for being frail. She requires assistance with activities of daily living and ambulation and is eating-dependent. She has diagnoses of Parkinson's disease, hypertension, vascular dementia, mild depression, and multimorbidity, and is receiving psychological services.

Medical record notes dated April 20, 2010 document that *M* is receiving comfort care, followed by a May 5, 2010 note that *M* was recertified for hospice care in this period but might not meet hospice criteria in the next period. *M* was discharged from hospice care in July 2010. After discharge from hospice, *M* was referred to physical therapy to maximize her level of functioning and reduce the burden of care on nursing staff, as documented in the medical record. A physical therapy evaluation in October 2010 documents that *M* reached maximum potential. She remains confined to a wheelchair and is unable to stand without assistance.

M has decision-making capacity and makes her own decisions. The Social Work Department identified *M* as a resident with decision-making capacity. There is no documentation in the medical record of a clinical assessment of incapacity by a physician.

M's daughter attended the annual care planning meeting on June 10, 2010. Quarterly meetings are usually held without the resident and family unless there is a particular concern or issue that has to be addressed. *M*'s plan of care is discussed at these meetings. *M*'s social worker reported that *M* voiced concerns at one meeting that on one or two days she did not have breakfast. The nurse practitioner is the member of the team who is responsible for explaining to *M* any changes in her medical care or status, such as eligibility for or discharge from hospice.

There is documentation in the medical record that *M* makes her own medical decisions about her care at care planning meetings. Her social worker reports that her daughters do not make decisions for her. She lets them know, "I am the mother." The social worker also reports that *M* did participate in discussions about her admission and discharge from hospice. A July 16, 2010 social work note documents that the family was informed of changes in *M*'s plan of care when *M* was discharged from hospice on July 14, 2010.

M was assessed as stable at her August 2010 quarterly review. Neither the resident nor the family participated in the quarterly review.

2. *Case findings*

This case involves a frail elderly woman, whom we shall refer to as *M*, who was enrolled and disenrolled from hospice while residing in the long-term care unit of a nursing home. In interviews with *M*, *M* describes her relationships with her daughter whom she appointed as her health care agent. She also reveals that she is not comfortable with her participation in the care planning and decision process that led to her enrollment and disenrollment in hospice. She describes her lived experiences in becoming a hospice patient at the nursing home and the limitations that she met with as a result of this change. One of her primary concerns is her inability to walk and loss of function, and the discontinuation of physical therapy when she became a hospice patient. She expresses strong emotion about this change in her care and her consistent failure to be able to access these services that she sees as critical to her health and well being.

The data show *M*'s engagement in end-of-life planning and the patient decision making process, and openness to such processes. Patient decision making for *M* is a process that is ongoing, changes over time and is multidimensional. It includes decisions about health care treatment as well as other decisions about *M*'s person-centered care needs, such as whom she trusts to make decisions for her when she no longer has capacity, and future planning decisions. And it is a process that is both social because it involves social systems in which *M* is embedded such as family and provider, and is self-directed, driven by self-agency. Patient decision making for *M* is characterized by a high degree of self-control, self-efficacy and agency, and involves cognitive, affective, social, and cultural dimensions.

M shares that she has a DNR Order and a Health Care Proxy. *M*'s engagement in forms of end-of-life planning is a decision process in itself and involves desire and agency. But what distinguishes the end-of-life planning decision process from everyday decision making is the goal toward which *M* directs her agency—her own end of life. She embraces that the horizon structure of suffering in end-of-life decision making has an end of life in a futural horizon about which she can make decisions in the present.

One of those decisions is the appointment of her daughter as the person she trusts to make decisions for her and *"take charge"* of everything. She has also had meaningful conversations with her daughter about end-of-life options such as feedings tubes and burial arrangements. The centrality of communication to *M*'s relational meanings and conversations is salient in the end-of-life planning discussions she has with her daughter. The choices and decisions *M* makes depend on her being able to communicate those choices and decisions effectively to her daughter, whom she has appointed to be her health care agent and to act for her when she no longer has capacity. The trust she has in her daughter and their relational intimacy found the type of communication they have—the good conversations. Therefore, there is also valuing involved in patient decision making. *M* attaches value attributes to her decision process and her decision outcomes.

M describes the experiences she lived through with her two husbands who died of cancer, and her brother to whom she remained faithful, "foot-to-foot," until his death. In recalling these past experiences, she is expressing her end-of-life wishes about her own future care planning in her current situation in the nursing home, and about the kind of care, attention, and fidelity she expects from her relational caregivers. In discussing her burial arrangements, she discusses freely the hymns she has thought about. She shows no discomfort in having these discussions about the end of life or engaging in the complex thought and decision-making processes involved in forgoing treatment.

M appeals to her caregiver to rub ointment on her back to relieve the soreness and burning she is experiencing. This is an example of *M*'s coping with her suffering condition through decision making about her care, a manifestation of her agency. The example shows that her decision has the meaning of an attempt to restore empathic care and, through it, embodied comfort and security, to eliminate the detrimental aspects of the world, that is, burning pain.

The decision to forgo cardiopulmonary resuscitation in the event of cardiac arrest reflects *M*'s agentic processes at work in end-of-life decision making. Forgoing treatment is a complex decision process because it involves choosing between two alternative treatments, weighing the risks, benefits, and burdens of each treatment, deliberating about the alternatives, and making a judgment. In this process, *M*'s end of life becomes thematic for her. *M* evaluates the burden to herself, the patient, of prolonging life through life-sustaining treatment that is likely to heighten her suffering and be a burden to relational others. She also evaluates the alternative of refusing life-sustaining treatment, choosing to have a natural death that is unassisted by medical technology, and that may assure her relief from the burden of suffering in a futural horizon. She gives testimony that she does not wish to be a burden to her family.

The concept of burden has complexity in the end-of-life decision making process that discloses itself in the data as having social and relational dimensions.

I.   RELATIONSHIPS WITH HEALTH CARE PROFESSIONALS

M's relationships with her health care professionals and direct care staff at the nursing home are part of her situatedness in the nursing home community and environment, and the social context of elder decision making. Overall, *M* does not have highly developed relationships with the professionals or staff. This is particularly devastating for her given the relational discontinuity she has experienced with family members after her traumatic displacement from her home. She does not express confidence in her doctor, psychologist, or spiritual care professionals, and cites infrequent conversations with her social worker. The relational problems that she experiences weaken the communication between *M* and the staff. Her response to her hospice admission and discharge is emblematic of these relational and communication inconsistencies. As a result of these inconsistencies that rupture *M*'s perceptions of self-efficacy, she does not turn to these relationships in the context of decision making.

II.   TYPES OF HEALTH CARE DECISIONS

There are three types of treatment decisions in which *M* is involved in the nursing home: (i) decisions which involve routine health care such as medications for pain; (ii) decisions which involve functioning such as physical therapy services, and (iii) major treatment decisions such as changes in the goals of care that are related to the trajectory of *M* illnesses. *M*'s concern with the various types of health care decisions in her life in the nursing home relate to her sense of health and well being. One type of decision and self-care is those involving everyday choices and deliberations, such as seeking medication for pain or soothing ointment for irritated and raw skin.

While certain areas of everyday decision making could be viewed as routine, as they involve regular care needs, the participant's experience of the illness or the care need cannot be described as routine. A good example of this is *M*'s experience of pain, such as the pain she describes in her knees and in her hands. While *M*'s pain level is assessed as "none" or "controlled" as documented in the medical record, her communication of her pain experience appears not to be consistent with this assessment. There is a moral claim for relief of pain made by *M* who presents in pain, showing her pained hands and limbs. In that sense, independent of its intensity and quality, assessment and treatment of any pain are not routine. Abandonment of the resident in a state of pain heightens the resident's pain and leads to suffering.

Other types of routine decisions in which *M* is involved are decisions that affect her functional level. *M* experiences perhaps the most anguish about her health care as that care relates to her functional decline in ambulation.

This concern is directly related to the discontinuation of physical therapy by the nursing home staff during the period documented in the medical record prior to discharge from hospice. In view of *M*'s burning desire to walk and to achieve mobility, this discontinuation of physical therapy services is greeted by *M*. with terrible frustration and anger. She also expresses persistent unhappiness that she felt she was not made a part of the care planning conversations that led to this decision to terminate her physical therapy services.

This issue has meaning for *M* in terms of the resident decision-making process and communication. She feels that not only has she suffered relational losses, but these losses have been compounded by communication failures. *M* experiences a connection between interpersonal relations and communication. For her, relationality founds communication; weak interpersonal relationships appear to limit effective communication between the resident and her health care professionals. In this context, decision making and its constitutive processes of deliberation and practical evaluation are revealed as expressions of agency. *M* draws upon this powerful sense of agency in the process of decision making involving her health care professionals at the nursing home, which she experiences as giving her very little voice in making decisions about her care.

III.   ADMISSION AND DISCHARGE FROM HOSPICE

A major health care decision for *M* in the nursing home is both the admission to and discharge from hospice. *M* communicates a weak sense of agency about the decision to be enrolled in hospice, and about the decision to be discharged when she gains weight, begins to flourish and is no longer eligible for hospice services. This means that she does not seem to comprehend fully the nature of the decisions made and her authorship of the decision process. She suggests that she did not participate fully in the decision process. The decision was presented to her as a *fait d'accompli* or factual state of affairs. However, she is by no means passive or non-agentic. She does share that she was told post facto that she was on hospice and has tried to adjust to this change, and to accept that this is probably the best path for her at this stage of her illness. Throughout her hospice stay, however, she has struggled to make herself a decision maker by reflecting on and challenging her post-decision state of affairs.

M questions why she is not receiving physical therapy services and protests the inability of her hospice aide to assist her with walking. *M* has a passionate desire to walk and will not allow her desire to be extinguished by her enrollment in hospice. She persists in questioning why she is not receiving physical therapy services and why she did not participate more fully in the decision-making process for her to go on hospice. *M* does not understand the role of the hospice aide and experiences a high level of exasperation that her intention to achieve mobility is not enabled. Communication emerges as a theme in the data with respect to this major decision. In the excerpt below,

M describes her "story" of finding out that she has a hospice aide, and what that means to her:

> Excuse me a little...what's her name now, S—[the hospice aide]? So ... that's—I told S—to let—S—is the girl that you all paid to sit here with me, right? S—sits with me. Oh, you didn't know about it, too? Well, I don't know. They didn't put it through me. It was after they finished, they tell me that they pick a girl to come in early in the morning and sit with me and if I want anything upstairs, she [S—] could do that.
> My daughter was involved in the decision. I think so. Because I wasn't there. No. So the details, I don't know, but she's [S] supposed to come in and, when I left, she's supposed to make the bed and straighten up the room. So, that's as much as I could tell you about it. So...I haven't spoken to anybody. Anyway.
> No, I only heard the name "hospice." But not anybody tell me anything. Because I was even kind of scared to hear the word hospice and—but now I am getting accustomed here ... and don't tell anybody that I am around hospice. They say, "Mammy, that's the best—that's the best for you because you know we don't have anybody at home to stay with you and I am afraid when you cook, you might leave the gas on." So that's why I am here. So that's my story.

The decision to be assessed for and enrolled in hospice care is a major change in goals of care for *M*. But *M* makes very clear that this was a decision process from which she felt distanced, isolated, and minimally involved. She was told of the decision after she was enrolled in hospice when she is introduced to S, her hospice aide. *M* also describes the involvement of her daughter, her health care agent, in the decision. In this description of the surrogate's role in the decision process, there arises a tension between ethical principles of autonomy and beneficence.

M no doubt believes that her daughter-surrogate acted in her best interest, as indicated by the story she narrates, but her daughter's assessment of her best interests appears to conflict with *M*'s desire to be autonomous.

M understands what hospice is and, although she confesses that at first it frightened her, she has grown "accustomed" to her new role as a hospice patient. Because her family tells her that the decision is in her best interest and she can no longer function independently, she attempts to take up the role of the hospice patient and reframe her autonomy in a relational context.

However, *M* does not fully accept the consequences of the change in her goals of care. S, the hospice aide, does not meet *M*'s expectations in terms of how she understands her goals of care. *M* had a strong desire to walk and expected that the hospice aide would assist her in achieving her goals to improve her functioning. This did not happen and caused *M* great distress. This disconnect between *M*'s expectations for the hospice aide and *M*'s care needs reflects both a fundamental misunderstanding about hospice care on *M*'s part, and a relational communication breakdown on the part of the health care professionals and the interdisciplinary team to the extent they failed to discuss with *M* and help her understand her goals of care and care preferences, and how those preferences would be translated into medical orders. *M* accepted hospice only insofar as it meant to her that she was possibly becoming increasingly frail and approaching the end of life, but she did not translate the meaning of hospice on a practical level into the outcome that she would no longer receive assistance with her ambulation or would have a significant decline in functioning.

When hospice is discontinued, similarly, *M* is not informed of the change in goals of care. *M* is not able to exercise any self-determination or control. This surrendering of autonomy in patient decision making and diminution of perceptions of self-efficacy are forms of suffering for *M* in the nursing home environment.

3.   *Discussion and analysis*

There are several key questions that emerge from the above case study and findings that relate directly to the role of the surrogate in health care decision making at the end of life, and the role and value of the surrogate. They are:

- What is the responsibility of the surrogate when a resident has fluctuating capacity?
- Who is the decision maker?
- When does the surrogate have legal responsibility to act?
- What is the ethical relation of the surrogate to the resident and what moral obligations arise in the absence of legal authority to make decisions?
- How does the surrogate negotiate her own values and give life and meaning to the values and preferences of resident? Does this process involve only substituted judgment, or evaluation of suffering?
- What is the role of the nursing home and nursing home staff?
- What is the role of the nursing home ethics committee?

I. CAPACITY ISSUES

This case raises very significant issues about the role of surrogates, and the health care professionals who support them, in relation to frail elderly persons who may have fluctuating capacity. This particular case falls under the law of New York State, which is clear in setting forth the requirements for clinical assessment of capacity and determination of incapacity by physicians. Unless there is a determination of incapacity by a physician with a concurrence by a second physician under the New York State Health Care Proxy Law, a patient is presumed under the law to have capacity to make decisions.

Assessment of capacity is task-specific, and a nursing home resident's capacity may fluctuate over time, even short periods of time. There is a relationship between the complexity of the decision and the level of capacity needed to make a decision. For example, the same level of capacity required to make a major medical treatment decision is not needed to appoint a health care agent under the New York State Health Care Proxy law, as the decision is not as complex. In the presenting case, there is no documentation of a determination of incapacity in the record. The social work staff of the nursing home communicate that the resident has decision making capacity. Even more compellingly, the resident's social worker describes the resident's sense of personal empowerment, her reluctance to have family members make any decisions for her, and her strong voice in communicating with nursing home staff in order to have her needs met. One example shared is the resident's negotiation with staff about her food choices, and her request to have the staff make tea for her.

While the medical record does document that the resident has vascular dementia, it appears to be in its early stages and according to all reports, does not interfere with the resident's ability to make health care decisions. No assumptions can be made that because the resident has early-stage dementia, the resident does not have decision making capacity. Residents or patients with dementia can still have task-specific decision-making capacity.

II. LEGAL AND ETHICAL RESPONSIBILITIES OF SURROGATE

In light of the resident's medical information and medical and social history, it is clear that the resident is the decision maker and exercises autonomy and self-determination about her care choices and decisions. It is the legal and ethical responsibility of the surrogate, in this case the resident's daughter who is the health care agent, to honor the wishes of the resident. The resident describes in some depth the trust she holds in her daughter, how she values this trust deeply and what it means to her. The surrogate is called upon to treat the trust invested in her with the highest respect.

Ethically, the surrogate also has a moral responsibility to spend time having conversations with the resident whose care has been entrusted to the surrogate, and seek to understand as well as possible what the resident's values and preferences are about her future care. If the surrogate feels it necessary and has the permission of the resident, he or she may also seek the help and support of the nursing home staff in the conversation process. However, it is only when there is a determination of incapacity that the authority of the surrogate is legally effective to make decisions on behalf of the resident, who is then incapable of making decisions on her own. A determination of incapacity was never made in this case, and therefore the health care agent had no legal authority to make health care decisions on behalf of the resident.

An important point that emerges from these case findings is that the legal and ethical responsibilities of the surrogate are not co-extensive with each other. In this case, the surrogate is the appointed health care agent who has no legal authority to make health care decisions because there has been no determination of incapacity. However, as an appointed health care agent, even in the absence of such effective legal authority, there arise moral obligations to the resident. The health care agent stands in ethical relation to the resident and must take active steps to carry out her fiduciary role and responsibilities. What is the nature of that role and responsibility? Is it contractual?

We reject the notion that the surrogate's value to the resident is a social contract or solely transactional in nature. Instead, we argue that the surrogate's value to the resident or patient is fundamentally social and relational. Drawing upon the work and writing of French philosopher and phenomenologist Emmanuel Levinas (1969), we recognize a pre-ontological and pre-theoretical moral claim that the patient makes upon the surrogate, which the surrogate cannot deny or refute. Westphal (2008) has described this claim as "heteronomous subjectivity." However, we depart from a strict construction of Levinasian philosophy in acknowledging the presence of reciprocity in the relationship between the resident and the surrogate. While the presence of such reciprocity is not in the nature of a *quid pro quo* or transactional exchange, and further does not, as Levinas feared, vitiate the value of the ethical relation, reciprocity that arises in the ethical relation is part of a recovery process for the suffering, seriously ill individual whose capacity to give to another is a self-affirming, agentic and healing intentional movement and act (Davidson & Shahar, 2007; Davidson & Cosgrove, 2008). Throughout *M*'s interviews, *M* reveals a capacity to be relational, giving, and loving toward her daughter and her family, even as she suffers cascading losses.

III.   HONORING WISHES, VALUES, AND PREFERENCES OF RESIDENT

The critical question in this case becomes how the surrogate should have carried out her ethical responsibilities in a way that would have honored the wishes, values and preferences of the resident. The resident expressed a powerful sense of trust in her daughter, whom she appointed as her health care agent. She turned to her daughter over and over again when she experienced frustration in dealing with the nursing home and the nursing home staff, and when she felt her needs were not being met in the way she expected or desired. Yet in the most major decisions of *M*'s serious illness involving her admission and discharge from hospice, the evidence seems to indicate that her daughter was not her advocate in the decision-making process at the nursing home. Somehow, *M,* who was the decision maker, was marginalized. The surrogate in this case appears to have substituted her own values and judgment for the frail elderly resident's and without specific legal authority, violating the fiduciary relation. Even if there were a grant of legal authority, the standard of substituted judgment means exactly the opposite—making decisions based upon what the patient would have wanted.

In the absence of legal authority to act, what could or should the surrogate have done to advocate on her mother's behalf? First, she should have made it very clear to the nursing home staff that all care planning conversations were to be held with her mother, as her mother was the decision maker. She should have taken steps herself, and with the help of the social work staff, to assure that her mother received the help she needed to understand what her care options were and what those options meant: the risks and the benefits, and the alternatives. If these conversations had occurred employing skilled communication strategies, *M* would have better understood what she was giving up by going on hospice and what care she would be receiving that she had not had access to before. Perhaps *M* would have decided that hospice was not the right option for her in light of her goals of care, and that non-hospice palliative care was an acceptable alternative. And most importantly, *M*'s surrogate could and should have taken an active role in reducing her mother's illness burden and preventing and relieving her pain and suffering. The ethical responsibility of the surrogate surpasses understanding of the seriously ill individual's wishes, values and preferences. It is incumbent upon the surrogate to evaluate and relieve the suffering burden of the resident.

This case provides a very rich understanding of the complexities of decision making for a seriously ill individual at the end of life, and the ethical role and responsibilities of the surrogate who stands in ethical relation to the resident or patient. We learned that the surrogate's relation of trust to the resident is not co-extensive with the grant of legal authority. Moral obligations to the resident arise with the investment of trust in the surrogate. The surrogate is valued because he or she is trusted and is called upon to serve the suffering individual and relieve that suffering.

C. Recommendations

This case study and findings highlight the importance of education for surrogates and interdisciplinary professionals about the role and legal and ethical responsibility of surrogates, especially in addressing ethical dilemmas that arise in connection with the exercise of their responsibilities to seriously ill older persons whose care has been entrusted to them. This is a priority area of education in both ethics and end-of-life care that has not received sufficient attention and constitutes a barrier to policy implementation. For professionals, education that helps to develop knowledge and skill competencies in care coordination and communication, including assessment and empathic listening and providing social and emotional support to surrogates, is critical.

At the systems level, a heightened focus on improving communication and initiating earlier conversations with seriously ill older persons through shared informed decision-making processes that involve surrogates even before they have a grant of legal authority, with the permission of the resident or patient, will help to avoid conflict at the end of life. Such process conversations can help older persons who are seriously ill or at end of life dwell more deeply and amplify their discussions about goals of care and their wishes, values, and preferences, and as appropriate have goals of care translated into medical orders. Social workers have a pivotal role to play in both initiating and advancing these conversations and negotiating conflict that may arise among older persons and their surrogates and interdisciplinary team members.

Finally, affirming the dignity of the suffering human person in serious illness at the end of life and the person's capacity for human agency, human development and freedom to act and make choices and decisions, sometimes even in states of disability and dementia, is a core value of ethics in the exercise of surrogate responsibility.

III.   Ethics committees and ethics committee education

The architects of the New York Family Health Care Decisions Act (2010) wisely saw that it would be prudent to obligate all nursing homes and hospitals covered under the law to establish ethics review committees. While many health care facilities already had such committees in place prior to enactment of the law, such a provision in state law established an authoritative function of the ethics review committee. However, comprehensive education for committee members in a number of critical areas is essential to the proper functioning of such ethics review committees.

Importantly, there is growing research evidence that many aging and health professionals today lack adequate training in ethics, as well as in palliative and end-of-life care, both in and outside the United States. A recent report issued by the Lien Foundation (Murray, 2015) ranking palliative care across the world puts the United States at ninth among 80 countries, based upon measures of quality and availability of palliative care. The Lien Foundation white paper also addresses in more depth the continuum of sociological, cultural and ethical issues that affect end-of-life care. One of the key recommendations in the report is the centrality of capacity building and training to the growth of palliative and end-of-life care, not only for physicians, nurses and other aging and health professionals, but for community-based volunteers, caregivers and surrogate decision makers.

Palliative care both as a philosophy of care and as a delivery system is a meaningful context for understanding processes of ethical decision making, both for older adults and their surrogates. Consistent with this context, it would be important to include content on applicable state laws governing decision making and palliative care in ethics committee and interprofessional education and training.

A.   Core curricula areas for ethics review committee education

There are several critical areas that should be included in a comprehensive educational curriculum for ethics review committees:

• Introduce foundational content on the existing legal and ethical consensus for decision making, and the principles and goals of palliative care.

- Explain the paradigm shift in health care decision making framework, relevance to interdisciplinary team process and communication skill competencies of team members.
- Describe the paradigm shift in functions of the ethics review committee as defined under state law, committee process and procedures specific to the ethics review committee, and responsibilities of ethics review committee members.
- Provide targeted overview of key provisions of state laws, including decision making standards, applicable facility policies on health care decision making, and implementation challenges.
- Discuss the role and responsibility of the ethics review committee in addressing conflict and assisting in resolving conflict.
- Formulate consensus about adoption of best practice to assure ethically competent functioning of the ethics review committee, and consultation and communication with family members, surrogates, and health care professionals.

While it is not possible to address each of these areas exhaustively, we touch upon the central purpose of the education in each core area. In developing or modifying an educational curriculum to find the best "fit" for the particular facility and ethics review committee being trained, certain decisions will have to be considered in consultation with the leadership of the committee or the parties who have requested the training. One important decision is whether the training should be presented in one, two or multiple modules or sessions. This decision may depend on facility resources and availability of, or access to, committee members. The second decision is to determine the time and resources that should be invested in developing written curricula for the training program. Certain parts of the written curricula may be standardized, but other parts may be facility-dependent. It is advised, however, that there be written curricula materials developed and provided to the ethics review committee members to supplement the training that will be presented to them based upon the core educational curricula.

A third decision is whether to include an interdisciplinary professional or professionals from a mix of disciplines in the training program. It is frequently very helpful to incorporate such an interdisciplinary perspective and have representation from more than one discipline in conducting training programs, especially for a body such as an interdisciplinary ethics review committee.

1.   Legal and ethical consensus: Principles and goals of palliative care

State law provisions may address the composition of ethics review committees. Hospitals and nursing facilities may be required to have a written policy that has provisions addressing ethics review committee composition. While the provisions of state law may impose certain prescriptive requirements on hospitals and nursing homes, such as interdisciplinarity and number of health and social services practitioners, covered institutions may still exercise certain discretion in terms of how they draft their policy provisions on committee membership, operationalize the applicable requirements, and form or restructure the membership of committees. For this reason, committee members will likely have very diverse backgrounds, knowledge and training in ethics and health care decision making.

It is critical that professionals who are developing educational curricula for ethics committee members not take for granted that all individual members of the committee have a working knowledge of essential constituents of the existing legal and ethical consensus about decision making under applicable federal and state laws and regulations, as well as broadly accepted consensus statements on ethical aspects of treatment decisions issued by national or state bodies such as statements on palliative sedation. It is always helpful to have a sense of the knowledge level among the individuals being trained. Frequently, however, that will not be possible. In this introductory segment of the training, it is appropriate to define the objectives of the training and integrate the broad goals of palliative care with those objectives.

Participants in the training should be made aware of state laws on palliative care and decision making, and how statutory provisions and requirements intersect with existing law. Consistent with the work of Joseph J. Fins (2006), who framed the overarching heuristic of a palliative ethic of care, it is imperative to spend time in the training session describing the principles and goals of palliative care in enhancing quality of life, relieving suffering, fostering effective communication and supporting person-centered decision making. This education is critical to helping committee members understand the connections in palliative care between interdisciplinary team practice, communication and good decision making. This context will provide committee members with a heightened awareness and sensitivity to the limits of the medical futility principle in resolving conflicts at the bedside and foster a more humanistic attitude toward working with suffering family members and addressing their ethical concerns. Committee members should be provided with literature on palliative care, or, at a minimum, references to resources that provide information about palliative care, such as the National Consensus Project for Quality Palliative Care and the Center to Advance Palliative Care at the Mount Sinai School of Medicine, New York City.

Following a discussion of the goals of palliative care, it would be important to review at least briefly certain key points of the existing legal and ethical consensus in the areas of advance care planning, resident/patient/elder rights, informed consent and decision making, refusal of treatment, life-sustaining treatment, withholding and withdrawal of life-sustaining treatment, pain and symptom management, and palliative sedation (including some of the defined terms under the statutes), in an effort to put everyone on the same page. As it is unlikely that time constraints will permit a comprehensive review of this information, written materials should be provided to the committee members in each of these areas referencing applicable law and applicable consensus statements of appropriate bodies.

2. *Paradigm shift: Relational framework in decision making*

In the years following the *Cruzan* (1990) decision, and the enactment of the federal Patient Self-Determination Act of 1990 and state health care proxy laws, policy making in the area of health care decision making has been driven in large part by the patient rights movement. The legal and ethical underpinnings for such policy making have been based on well-established ethical principles of patient autonomy and health care justice. However, the rational choice, self-interested agency and transactional pillars of the individualistic framework have been challenged on a number of fronts as inadequate and not sufficiently accommodating cultural differences in decision making, social, ecological and community contexts, and the multidimensional aspects of person-centered decision making—psychological, cognitive, emotional, spiritual, axiological. The movement away from a contractarian, formalistic approach, and toward a more relational framework of decision making, marks the next era in the ethics of health care decision making. This shift reflects the humanistic perspective that persons are fundamentally social and relational, and that rights are relational. It also challenges the widely held notion that health care decision making has only epistemological foundations.

Turning to New York as an example, the enactment of the FHCDA in New York is consistent with this paradigm shift. The statute formally recognizes in law the well-established social and ethical role and responsibilities of families and family members as relational others and in many cases, as caregivers, in the health care decision-making process. It is long overdue that this role be given legal status and legitimacy in our statutes, policies and systems of decision making. Ethics committee members need to be introduced to the relational framework in decision making and its essential constituents: the interpersonal relationship, communication that is founded on relationality, moral agency and responsibility, and collaborative practice. This education should be integrated into a description of the role of the interdisciplinary team in clinical settings, and the relevance of the paradigm to effective functioning of the interdisciplinary team at the specific facility.

The last component of the education in this core area that should be touched upon is to expose committee members to some understanding of the complexity that is involved in any decision-making process across systems. Briefly, the levels of decision making that should be identified are the microsystem in which the older person and the older person's experiences and interactions with family members, surrogate and personal support systems are situated; facility policies and systems; and the macrosystem external to the facility that influences such aspects of decision making as determination of government benefits and allocation of resources. Health care decisions usually involve interaction and communication across all system levels.

For example, a surrogate who is weighing a decision to withdraw or with-hold life sustaining-treatment for an older person who is terminally ill will be offered information and counseling from the older person's attending practi-tioner about palliative and end-of-life care options under state laws, such as referral to hospice and eligibility for the Medicare hospice benefit. There are multiple systems involved in the surrogate's decision-making process.

3.   *Paradigm shift: Function of ethics review committees*

In New York, the 2010 Family Health Care Decisions Act marks a paradigm shift not only in the role of families in decision making, but also in the role of ethics review committees in the decision-making process. The statute estab-lishes an authoritative function of the ethics review committee by investing it with legal authority to make binding decisions on certain matters. The tradi-tional consultative role of this committee is formalized under the statute. The statutory provisions explicitly stipulate that consistent with the functions of the ethics review committee, permitted responses to a matter it has reviewed may include advising, making a recommendation, or assisting in resolving a dispute about proposed health care. More specifically, however, the eth-ics review committee mandate under the statute is that it shall consider and respond to any matter submitted to it by a person connected with the case. This is a very broad mandate. The responsibility of ethics committee mem-bers to carry out this mandate has significant meaning for seriously ill older persons, their family members and surrogates.

The recommendations and advice of the committee shall be advisory and non-binding, except when a mandated review of a surrogate decision to with-hold or withdraw life-sustaining treatment is triggered. In these cases, the determination of the committee to approve or disapprove the decision with-holding or withdrawing life-sustaining treatment is binding. This new author-itative function of ethics committees requires much more extensive training for committee members to assure that they are properly qualified to carry out this weighty charge.

Explaining the complexity of decisions to forgo treatment, especially life-sustaining treatment, and the multilayered process of decision making involved in the choices and deliberations about treatments, risks, benefits and burdens, and alternative treatments, is a *sine qua non* of the training. Consistent with the relational paradigm of decision making, committee mem-bers will need to understand that their charge in reviewing surrogate deci-sions to withhold and withdraw life-sustaining treatment and issue a binding approval or disapproval of such decisions, is a responsibility that puts them in ethical relation to the elder resident/patient and the surrogate and ought not be taken lightly.

With respect to ethics committee process and procedures, the current pro-visions in the New York statute are skeletal. Facilities governed by the law need to have clearly delineated policies that address committee process and procedures. There is room for wide variation in terms of how the provisions of the statute can be operationalized. The training should cover the process and procedures of the specific facility policy as well as the statutory provisions, including respecting confidentiality of the committee process.

Members of the ethics committee should also be sensitized to the potential for conflicts of interest between professional codes of ethics for professionals in their respective disciplines represented on the committee, facility policies on health care decision making, or decisions made by the ethics review committee. This type of conflict is to be distinguished from conflicts of interest that arise due to a contractual relationship with the facility, or from conscience objections to treatment decisions made pursuant to the FHCDA. A decision on an ethical issue that presents a potential conflict for a social worker may not present a similar conflict for a physician or a nurse. The ethics of health care decision making and health care justice do not have a universal meaning for all professionals in all disciplines.

4.   *Targeted review of FHCDA and PCIA: Decision-making standards and patient rights*

The enactment of the FHCDA, while a positive and welcome step in New York, did add complexity to the health care decision-making process. In the larger framework of federal and state laws and regulations governing health care decision making, it is important to explain to ethics committee members how a law such as this one fits into the existing legal and regulatory scheme, as well as how it interacts with other laws, such as state palliative care laws. The focus of this review should be targeted to the scope of the law, surrogate selection, legal authority of the surrogate, informed decision making, and such areas of the statute that may give rise to conflict including capacity determinations, who is qualified under the statute and facility policy to make capacity determinations, and application of the clinical standards.

One of the most important areas of the training is the work that training professionals will need to conduct with ethics committee members to enable them to understand the decision-making standards. Under the FHCDA, there are two sets of standards: broad patient-centered standards and standards for life-sustaining treatment decisions. It is the second set to which trainers will need to turn their attention as these are not easy to understand, have been oversimplified in the first decade of the statute's implementation, and present significant implementation challenges. In addition, the trainers need to instruct ethics committee members that these standards do not mirror the standards for issuance of DNR Orders under Article 29-B of the New York Public Health Law, now repealed. The medical futility language in the old law has been eliminated from the new decision-making standards, in addition to other changes made.

In this chapter, it is impossible and impracticable to dissect these statutory standards in any depth. They are illustrative of the challenges practitioners face on the ground in implementing such standards and as a result, the kind of content that will need to be reviewed in depth with ethics committee members. First, the members of the committee must have some working familiarity with clinical terminology such as what is meant medically by an illness or injury which can cause death in six months, an irreversible or incurable condition, permanent unconsciousness, and withdrawal or withholding of life-sustaining treatment (a defined term in the statute). In addition, committee members must be instructed that there is no legal or ethical distinction between withdrawal and withholding of life-sustaining treatment, a central constituent of the existing legal and ethical consensus in health care decision making.

It is helpful in the training session to adopt a heuristic method by describing the life-sustaining treatment decision standards as being broken down into two "buckets." In each bucket, the standard has two parts that have to be parsed: an assessment of burden that will be made by the surrogate, and a clinical determination that will be made by the physician. Although the statute does not clearly define this line of demarcation, there is a working consensus among health care attorneys that this is how the standards should be implemented based upon legislative intent. There is no language in the statute that bars the surrogate and the physician from consultation; such consultation likely occurs in practice and should be encouraged to foster good communication and avoid disputes. There is also nothing in the statute that bars consultation with other members of the interdisciplinary team. Such consultation is also good practice.

Turning to the clinical determination first, it is helpful to present examples of clinical situations to ethics committee members and discuss whether the clinical criteria in either or both buckets would be met for the purpose of a surrogate decision to withdraw or withhold life-sustaining treatment. For example, a patient or resident who presents with diagnoses of congestive heart failure, coronary artery disease and advanced peripheral vascular disease is likely to meet the clinical criteria for an irreversible or incurable condition as determined by the attending physician with a physician concurrence, even though the patient may not be permanently unconscious or may not be expected to die within six months. Ethics review committee members serving in nursing homes will need to understand that decisions (other than CPR) made by surrogates in nursing homes that fall into the "neither terminally ill nor permanently unconscious" bucket are mandated reviews requiring a binding decision of the committee.

The second part of the analysis to walk the committee members through is how to parse the assessment of burden under the decision-making standards. This section of the statute may prove to be the biggest implementation challenge for surrogates, health care professionals and ethics committee members for a number of reasons. First, there has generally been a very narrow construction of what these standards mean, and a prevailing judgment among some health care professionals that they may be operationalized in the same way as the standards under the old DNR law. This is incorrect and would result in a serious denial of patient rights under the statute. These standards broaden the assessment of burden to the patient which needs to be made under the law. The medical futility language has been eliminated from the standards. Such a movement away from a medical futility standard for life-sustaining treatment decisions is a positive step, as medical futility by definition and in clinical practice means success or failure of a treatment, providing too limited a basis for weighing benefits and burdens to the patient. The medical futility standard under the old New York DNR law was never intended to serve as the basis of an assessment about quality of life.

More specifically, an entire reading of the FHCDA standards makes clear that the assessment of burden is a qualitative assessment, and one that takes into account the subjective experiences of the patient. Although in the first bucket the language of extraordinary burden does parallel the language of extraordinary burden in the old DNR law, the nature of the assessment is not tied to the patient's medical condition alone as it is in the old law. but involves a multidimensional assessment of the patient.

Similarly, the assessment of burden to the patient under the second bucket is qualitative and multidimensional, extending to pain, suffering or burden that would be experienced by the patient as inhumane or extraordinarily burdensome. Given the knowledge we are gaining every day about pain and the experience and meaning of pain to patients in serious illness, this inclusion within the statutory language of assessment of pain burden to the patient should be welcomed.

We know based upon research evidence that pain is often untreated and undertreated, and that uncontrolled, intolerable and intractable pain leads to suffering. Education provided to ethics committee members about what is involved in a multidimensional assessment of illness burden, pain and suffering under the provisions of the FHCDA will be critical to their proper and full review of matters that require provision of advice, recommendations and binding decisions.

5. A more humanistic response to conflict negotiation and resolution

One of the central roles of the ethics review committee is addressing conflict and assisting in the resolution of conflict. Conflict may arise within families or between health care professionals, or from communication breakdowns between the patient, family, surrogate and health care professionals. Facilities should have procedures in place to address and negotiate conflict informally through appropriate process. However, when conflict does reach the ethics review committee, the members of the committee need to have a foundation in understanding the relational dimensions of conflict, and the significant role communication plays in helping to resolve disputes. Research evidence suggests that communication is founded upon relation-centeredness. Therefore, education about the relational framework of decision making is likely to foster improved communication skills in dealing with conflict and a more humanistic, empathic response to conflict.

This is a core area of the educational curriculum that draws upon interdisciplinary knowledge and expertise in work with families. Sources of conflict in families may stem from distrust of the health care system, not receiving sufficient or well-explained information about the patient's diagnosis, prognosis, disease trajectory, or goals of care, and values differences. Palliative care and hospice have a well-known record of supporting distressed and grieving families in the decision-making process. And the interdisciplinary team in hospice is a model of collaborative practice that can be replicated in other clinical settings.

6.   Best practice and recommendations for research

In bringing to a close any training that may be provided to ethics committee members regardless of what it may have been possible to cover due to time constraints or other barriers, it would be important to help the group reach consensus about what is best practice in the particular facility for assuring ethically competent functioning of the ethics committee, and consultation and communication with family members, surrogates, and health care professionals.

We recommend that health care facilities and community-based and aging network agencies develop a research agenda that will support ethics committee functions through ongoing data collection and analysis that target measurement of outcomes. The implementation of state law provides a unique opportunity for aging and health professionals to collaborate with health care providers, in developing an evidence base that evaluates ethics training for ethics committee members and health care professionals working in health care settings, and the impact of such training on process and outcomes for patients. This type of evaluation should take place within the larger context of evaluating the impact of aging and health policy.

Professionals who are knowledgeable about state decision making and palliative care laws, and the principles discussed above, can make a significant contribution in providing comprehensive education and training to ethics review committees as part of the implementation of such laws, and restoring the centrality of ethics and collaborative practice to health care decision making and palliative care.

IV.   Conclusion

In this chapter, we examined New York health care decision making and palliative care laws as a case study in policy implementation, with a dual focus on the impact of such laws on older persons and systems. The experience of a frail, elderly nursing home resident in navigating decision processes related to transitions in care revealed the types of ethical dilemmas that may arise when an older person or nursing home resident has appointed a health care agent but may still have task-specific capacity to make certain decisions. The role of surrogate decision makers involves both legal and ethical responsibilities. These responsibilities may not be congruent in all cases and such incongruence may also not be well understood by the surrogate decision maker, or the members of the resident's interdisciplinary team. Surrogate decision makers may be in a unique position to serve as advocates for their capable loved ones with their consent, even though the surrogate decision maker may not have legal authority to make decisions. At all times, however, they must respect the limits of their legal authority.

Conflicts that cannot be resolved informally, or through the support of social work or the interdisciplinary team process, should be referred to the institutional ethics committee. Education for both surrogates and ethics committee members about palliative care, decision making and ethical dilemmas is critical to effective implementation of state palliative care and decision making laws and policy, and assuring that the rights, wishes, values and preferences of older persons are honored as part of the decision making process. Although this typically involves systems-level and cultural change and in most cases funding to support and sustain such change processes, it must be a priority. In addition, another type of much more far-reaching systems-level change would be choice architecture, such as if the structured decision-making of the hospice model of care were extended to non-hospice palliative care settings, effectively shifting the locus of default decision making to the system yet still permitting older persons or their surrogates to exercise full autonomy if those default decisions were not acceptable to them.

Acknowledgment

Portions of this chapter draw from the following works by Mary Beth Quaranta Morrissey:

Morrissey, M.B. (2012). Surrogate decision making: The surrogate's value. In K.J. Doka, A.S. Tucci, C.A. Corr, & B. Jennings (Eds), *End-of-life ethics: A case study approach* (pp. 62–83). Washington, DC: Hospice Foundation of America. Reprinted with permission from the Hospice Foundation of America.

Morrissey, M.B. (2011). Educating ethics review committees in a more humanistic approach to relational decision making. *New York State Bar Association Health Law Journal*, *16*(1). Reprinted with permission from: *Health Law Journal*, Spring 2011, *16*(1), published by the New York State Bar Association, One Elk Street, Albany, NY 12207.

References

Bullock, K. (2011). The influence of culture on end-of-life decision making. *Journal of Social Work in End-of-Life and Palliative Care, 7*(1), 83–98.

Centers for Medicare & Medicaid Services (2016). *Reform of requirements for long-term care facilities: Comprehensive person-centered care planning,* 42 C.F.R. § 483.21.

Cruzan v. Director, Missouri Department of Health. 497 U.S. 261 (1990).

Davidson, L., & Shahar, G. (2007). From deficit to desire: A philosophical reconsideration of action models of psychopathology. *Philosophy, Psychiatry, And Psychiatry, 14*(3), 215–232.

Davidson, L., & Cosgrove, L. (2008). Psychologism and phenomenological psychology revisited, part II: The return to positivity. *Journal of Phenomenological Psychology, 33,* 2141–2177.

Dijulio, B., Hamel, L., Wu, B., & Brodie, M. (2017). *Serious illness in late life: The public's view and experiences.* Menlo Park, CA: Kaiser Family Foundation.

Fins, J.J. (2006). *A palliative ethic of care: Clinical wisdom at life's end.* Sudbury, MA: Jones and Bartlett.

Gutheil, I.A., & Heyman, J.C. (2005). Communication between older people and their health care agents: Results of an intervention. *Health & Social Work, 30*(2), 107–116.

Halpern, N.A., Pastores, S.M., Chou, J., Chawla, S., & Thaler, H.T. (2011). Advance directives in an oncologic intensive care unit: A contemporary analysis of their frequency, type and impact. *Journal of Palliative Medicine, 14*(4), 483–489.

Institute of Medicine (IOM). (2015). *Dying in America: Improving quality and honoring individual preferences near the end of life.* Washington, DC: National Academies Press.

Levinas, E. (1969). *Totality and infinity: An essay on exteriority.* Pittsburgh, PA: Duquesne University Press.

Meisel, A. (2003). The legal consensus about forgoing life-sustaining treatment: Its status and its prospects. *Kennedy Institute of Ethics Journal, 2*(4), 309–345.

Morrissey, M.B. (2011). Phenomenology of pain and suffering: A humanistic perspective in gerontological health and social work. *Journal of Social Work in End-of-Life and Palliative Care, 7*(1), 14–38.

Morrissey, M.B., & Jennings, B. (2006, Winter). A social ecology of health model in end-of-life decision-making: Is the law therapeutic? *New York State Bar Association. Health Law Journal. Special Edition: Selected Topics in Long-Term Care Law, 11*(1), 51–60.

Murray, S. (2015). *The 2015 quality of death index: Ranking palliative care across the world.* New York: Economist Intelligence Unit Lien Foundation.

New York Public Health Law, Art. 29-B. (1988). Orders not to resuscitate for people in mental hygiene facilities.

New York Public Health Law, Art. 29-C. (1990). Health care agents and proxies.

New York Public Health Law Art. 29-CC. (2010).

New York Public Health Law, §2997-c. (2011).

New York Public Health Law, §2997-d. (2011).

Nicholas, L.H., Langa, K.M., Iwashyna, T.H., & Weir, D.R. (2011). Regional variation in the association between advance directives and end-of-life Medicare expenditures. *Journal of the American Medical Association, 306*(13), 1447–1453.

Patient Protection and Affordable Care Act, Pub. L. No. 111-148, 124 Stat. 119–1025 (2010). Retrieved December 14, 2017 from: www.gpo.gov/fdsys/pkg/PLAW -111publ148/content-detail.html

Patient Self-Determination Act of 1990, Pub. L. No. 101–508. (1990).

Rogers, C.R. (1961). *On becoming a person.* Boston, MA: Houghton-Mifflin.

Sabatino, C., & Karp, N. (2011). *Improving advanced illness care: The evolution of state POLST programs.* Washington, DC: AARP Public Policy Institute.

SUPPORT Principal Investigators. (1995). A controlled trial to improve care for seriously ill hospitalized patients: The study to understand prognoses and preferences for outcomes and risks of treatments (SUPPORT). *Journal of the American Medical Association, 274,* 1591–1598.

Wennberg, J.E., Fisher, F., Goodman, D.C., & Skinner, J. (2008). *Tracking the care of patients with severe chronic illness: The Dartmouth atlas of health care 2008.* Lebanon, NH: Dartmouth Institute for Health Policy and Clinical Practice.

Westphal, M. (2008). *Levinas and Kierkegaard in dialogue.* Indianapolis: Indiana University Press.

Part Four

Setting the stage for transforming elder care

9 Policy recommendations for more compassionate elder care

Systems reform, social justice, and sustainable social solidarity

> Wouldn't it be fitting if America had a truly great health system, with humane care throughout the life span? In the world's richest country, is it too much to ask that we treat everyone when they are sick, care for them when they are suffering, and allow them to die humanely and with dignity when the journey is over?
>
> (Professor Lawrence O. Gostin, *Milbank Quarterly*, December 2017)

I. Introduction

We open this concluding chapter of our book by calling attention to the question posed by eminent global public health law scholar Professor Lawrence O. Gostin in a recent op-ed in the *Milbank Quarterly* (2017). In this piece, Professor Gostin shares a moving account of his elderly father's recent experience negotiating the U.S. health system near the end of his life. After leading a rich and productive life as a worker, and a loving husband, father, grandfather, and great-grandfather, and at the ripe age of 101 years, Mr. Gostin found himself in a hospital that was unresponsive to his serious medical and psychosocial needs, as well as those of his family caregivers. In brief, Mr. Gostin was unable to access through the ordinary course the type of person- and family-centered palliative and supportive care that may have relieved his pain and suffering. Mr. Gostin's experience is that of every American. The question his son Larry Gostin poses is the right question at this time, and it invites thoughtful reflection upon our moral failing—one in which we all participate. It also demands urgent attention to the barriers that impede realization of the goals of humane systems of care for all Americans even in our last years and days, as well the design of possible responses and solutions.

We dare here to propose bold directions for aging and health policy, both in the United States and for the global society, in the next decades of the twenty-first century. In the case we make for policy reform, we acknowledge the ethical underpinnings of our arguments that rest upon recognition of the shared ethical obligation we owe to each and every older person—and to all members of society. We believe this ethical obligation is not restricted to the realm of theorizing, but is a felt, relational obligation to the suffering other in the encounter with the face of the suffering other (Levinas, 1969). The scope of issues we address in this book speaks to our attempt to paint a portrait of the suffering older adult, especially those older adults who are relegated to a marginal subsistence in the shadows of deprivation, poverty, inequity and injustice, and for whom there is no refuge. Through the nexus of the theoretical, practical, and ethical that we have traced in these book chapters, we ground a call for a collective commitment to radical social change and social action in the project to relieve suffering and improve life-course conditions of health and well being for all persons—from infancy through our very last days. In this last chapter, we bravely imagine a new social order that would rest upon major systems reforms, expansion of the social safety net and more just sharing of resources, mitigation of risks to our ecological home, and building of social bonds across all positions and generations.

II.   Portrait of growing old in America

Across all the chapters of this book, we have sketched in broad strokes a social ecology of aging at the various systems levels in which older persons are embedded. This social ecology of aging is closely aligned with a social ecology of suffering that transcends the boundaries of aging experience, but certainly encompasses many types of experiences older adults are living through, such as multimorbidity, functional limitations, impoverishment, trauma, displacement, and profound losses of home and community. In addition to these broad strokes, we have also shared accounts of older adults themselves encountering difficult realities in the health systems, such as Mrs. Zornow—mother of seven children—who had advanced dementia, nursing home resident *M* who was enrolled and discharged from hospice but felt marginalized in those care-planning and decision-making processes, and Mr. Gostin—loving husband, father, grandfather, and great-grandfather—who ended up in a hospital with acute medical needs but was given little information about his post-acute care options at discharge and as he neared the end of life. These older persons wouldn't fit well within the successful aging model that we discussed in Chapter 1. In the first instance, they were dealing with compromise, disability, and diminished reserves, which would make them outliers right off the bat under the successful aging constructs. On the other hand, it would not make sense to hold them personally accountable or responsible for the suffering they experienced in their later years, especially as their respective life changes and challenges were likely magnified and compounded by societal- and systems-level failures such as gaps in policy, knowledge, care, communication, and empathy. Echoing Larry Gostin, we ask what kind of society is it that would countenance indifference and cruelty to these frail elderly persons, who at one time were carers for others? It is doubtful that these were singular cases. May we then entertain the possibility that the highly touted "successfully aging" older adult, who eludes us in these examples, is a neoliberal construct that bears little relationship to reality? Based upon the massive body of evidence now available to us about aging, dying, and older adults themselves, we feel confident in taking the position that it's highly likely that the neoliberal, successful aging construct leaves at its margins certain populations of poor and vulnerable older persons among us, those with fewer resources and fewer years of education, and those who identify as members of racial-ethnic minority groups. No one has said it better than Olshansky and colleagues (2012), who have stated that the widening and persistent gap in health and longevity and increasing disparities have created "at least two 'Americas'" (p. 1803).

We would be remiss here if we did not mention economist Uwe Reinhardt (2012), whose critical commentaries and ideas resonate meaningfully with Gostin's and Olshansky's perspectives. Reinhardt's body of work suggests that the market-based health care system in America, with its roots in neoliberalism, is in essence class driven and has thus created inequities in access to health care through various forms of rationing, resulting in a tiered health care system. That tiered system makes it possible for those with resources to position themselves favorably to receive the best health care available in the United States, while permitting those with limited resources to suffer in conditions of impoverishment that are accompanied by other socially and economically determined states of health or illness, with little or no care. Even though Medicare has helped to reduce poverty among older adults, current rates are far higher than anyone would surmise—nearly half (45%) of adults ages 65 and older are living with incomes below 200% of the poverty thresholds as defined by the SPM in 2013 (compared to 33% of older adults under the official measure) (Cubanski, Casillas, & Damico, 2015). Even under the official measure, the rate of older adult poverty, magnified within demographic subgroups such as older women, older persons living alone, and racial and ethnic minority older persons, is unacceptably high. It is projected that proposals to privatize Social Security, raise premiums for Medicare, or drastically cut Medicare benefits and eviscerate entitlement programs would make older adults' crisis even more acute.

Failures to rescue older Americans from a future of poverty and marginalization rest not only with the market-based health care system, however, but with major failures in U.S. policy making. The biggest failure is unquestioningly the absence of any comprehensive long-term care policy in the United States or any central planning for long-term services and supports. Policy efforts at the state, local, and community levels can help to bridge some of these gaps, as Joanne Lynn has suggested in *MediCaring Communities* (2016), but can never make up entirely for the breadth and magnitude of the current void in federal policy making. From a historical perspective, in a little less than a 100 years, we have swung from the progressive policies of FDR's "New Deal" and Lyndon Baines Johnson's "Great Society," to the era of Reaganomics and neoliberalism beginning in the 1970s, and after eight years of Obamacare, a return to perhaps the most regressive policies that the United States has seen in its entire history. In very concrete and real terms, we continue to bear witness to the suffering of older adults who are hungry, who are homeless or do not have stable housing, who cannot get essential medical care and social services, and in many cases do not have the education or literacy to understand what their care options may be or how to navigate the aging and health systems. However, these experiences will pale next to the suffering we will witness during the Trump Era, and the serious threats to entitlement and welfare programs that stand in danger of being defunded and eviscerated. There is no doubt that U.S. policy failures in aging and health policy are very much moral failures not confined to the sphere of the market alone, with devastating implications for vulnerable older persons and their families and caregivers.

In her role as a nationally recognized social work educator, leader, and social justice advocate on behalf of vulnerable older persons, Mary Ann Quaranta made the remarkable observation in her later years, "Don't get old, but what's the alternative?" In this book, we have framed the aging public health crisis in terms of suffering, but always with careful attention to alternative models of care that would afford older persons possible opportunities for flourishing, resilience, and agency in the midst of suffering. We have offered public health strategies for shifting the market-based and transactional paradigm to elder-centered and palliative systems of care that will mitigate elder suffering. We make no bones about the radicality of this shift and what it involves in terms of the breadth of systems reforms, as well as social policy change, social action, and a cultural commitment to achieving equity, social justice, and a newly constituted social solidarity.

III.   Systems reform, social justice, and sustainable social solidarity

We propose a three-part framework and change agenda to address the salient gaps in aging, health policy, and systems: systems reform, social justice, and sustainable social solidarity.

A.   *Systems reform*

A public health systems perspective will be essential to aging and health systems transformation. That public health meta-framework must adopt a dual focus on infrastructure, and the social and economic determinants of health. Perhaps the worst kind of violence against vulnerable older persons is infrastructural violence—the inelasticity of our social and political structures and systems to respond meaningfully to older persons' overwhelmingly unmet needs. At the top of that pyramid of inequity is inequitable access to palliative care and pain relief. The World Health Organization has identified better palliative care for older persons as an urgent public health priority (Hall et al., 2011).

1.   Delivery system recommendations

To improve our delivery systems in a manner that is elder-centered will require structural changes that promote more systemic integration and coordination of care. As the consolidation process in health care evolves both vertically and horizontally, the emphasis should be shifted more heavily toward clinical and service integration rather than financial or business structures. With the concurrent evolution of information technology within health care, this will become ever more possible to accomplish independent of formal business structures, as these technologies enable us to overcome the siloed nature of EHR systems. Meanwhile, the role of the primary care physician (PCP) as the coordinator of care needs to be re-established, along with increased esteem and financial reimbursement to emphasize the important function that PCPs serve. This would have the added benefit of increasing the number of physicians and mid-level practitioners who choose primary care practices. In addition, it would reinforce the adoption of the Medical Home model, whose concepts and principles should become the expected norm for all of primary care. To the extent appropriate, these concepts could be expanded to medical and surgical specialties, which would facilitate smoother integration with the primary care Medical Home. Intrinsic to adoption of the Medical Home model across specialties would be a broader application of the team model to health care delivery, based on the premise that everyone should be positioned to function at the highest level of their license. Leveraging the team model across the health care spectrum would help to deliver the broader suite of services required for more complex chronic care, and partially mitigate the physician shortage that is projected amidst the growing demands of our elder population. Adoption of a true comprehensive team model would also include authenticating the older person's role in goals of care discussions, care planning, and decision making. The Medical Home also incorporates prevention and population management perspectives to complement the Hippocratic individual doctor-patient relationship and care model. These concepts should be adopted at all levels of medical care and synthesized with the individual doctor-patient relationship. Performance needs to be evaluated in a more balanced fashion, taking into account delivery of health care on an individual as well as population basis. All of these changes are aligned with the person- and family-centered palliative care model for older persons with serious illness, adopting a holistic focus on symptom relief and psychosocial needs, and informed by care-based personal values and individualized goals of care. The adoption and integration of these models of care would be synergistic and mutually reinforcing, with the relative contribution of each model determined by the severity of illness and needs and goals of the individual.

2.   Financing and reimbursement system reform

Financing and reimbursement models have a critical influence on the structures and outcomes of health care. Changes made to these systems should be directed towards the goal of producing valued outcomes reflecting better quality and efficiency for the entire population. If the United States is to establish "healthcare as a right," in providing equal access to vital health care services and reducing inequities in the current system, the government would need to establish a funding source and supporting insurance system adequate to ensure that the entire population has coverage for these basic services. This could be accomplished through expanded ACA funding for those individuals who are not supported under the current program, either through expansion of Medicaid eligibility or subsidies to make commercial insurance affordable for those not currently supported. The most radical option would be a shift to a single-payer model that utilizes the Medicare system to provide coverage of basic health care services, funded by the government, for all U.S. citizens. The single-payer model is operationally the simplest solution, but politically the most difficult.

Beyond the issue of access, further changes in the financing and reimbursement systems should be directed at the goal of supporting and reinforcing existing delivery models that are more integrated and coordinated, as well as other initiatives that would promote better quality and efficiency. The most important change in this direction is an accelerated transition from fee-for-service or transaction-based reimbursement to value- or performance-based models. This transition will better align incentives with improvements to health and elder care, focusing on and rewarding efforts that produce value for patients. Ideally, the performance goals should represent true outcome measures, not process measures or narrow quality goals that may or may not be correlated with better outcomes. Measuring and rewarding the performance of larger systems, in which patient population numbers are adjusted for severity of illness factors with a greater degree of statistical significance, eliminates the issues of statistical variation found with the small patient numbers associated with individual physicians and the potential for adverse selection of older and sicker patients. Evaluating multiple outcome factors for disease entities, and using broader measures for general health outcomes, helps to discourage siloed efforts that can produce unwanted outcomes in other aspects of a disease entity or a patient's overall health. This requires assessment of performance on a global population basis, as seen in global capitation models where an organization is responsible for quality and costs relating to an entire patient population, with the ability to direct its total revenue pool across the entire delivery system based on its determination of the best patient value, rather than arbitrary insurance or governmental rules and regulations. When the system is rewarded globally with appropriate sharing across the organization as a whole, this fosters the team effort necessary for optimal coordination and integration, allowing decisions to be made in the best interests of the older person and not considerations of income gain or loss, as currently witnessed between hospitals and physicians or specialists and primary care.

3. Psychosocial care and community-based models

The adoption of a comprehensive team model that honors the values and preferences of individuals often requires the integration of psychosocial support. While several standard-setting organizations have recognized the importance of social and emotional care as a part of their quality recommendations, there is more work to be done in this area. The emotional and practical concerns that older adults experience often affect how they cope with their illness. Integrating psychosocial support within models of care will ensure that older adults have the tools necessary to cope, explore their values and preferences, and receive guidance for communicating these to family members and medical teams.

The challenge of how to keep older adults healthy and safe when they are receiving services in the home is a critical one. Social isolation and reliance on family members and friends can be overwhelming, and ultimately unhealthy for older adults and their caregivers. Community-based nonprofits offer wrap-around ancillary services to patients and their families that can address any gaps in care. The landscape for new models of care is marked by innovation and collaboration, whether through interdisciplinary teams within organizations, or collaborations between community-based providers.

4. The promise of the public health approach to palliative care

We have devoted a good deal of space in the preceding chapters to the subject of palliative care because we are confident that this holds the greatest promise as a societal level and systems-level reform. The notions of palliative care for all, palliative care everywhere, and palliative care environments come closest to capturing the vision we have for embedding this kind of integrated care across all aging and health systems and in all units of the society. The Public Health Strategy for Palliative Care with its emphasis on policy development, implementation, education and training, as well as other WHO initiatives such as "Palliative Care for Older People: Better Practices" (Hall et al., 2011) and "Building Integrated Palliative Care Programs and Services" (Gomez-Batiste & Connor, 2017), will help to bridge the domains of medicine and social services. There is a growing consensus that a transition to integrated medical and social care—which can be implemented through such palliative care approaches—will be critical to systems transformation, as Joanne Lynn communicates so well in *MediCaring Communities*.

B. Social justice and equity: The preferential option for the poor

A recent article in *The New Yorker* (Levy, 2017), profiling Ophelia Dahl and her work in global public health, draws attention to "the preferential option for the poor," a social justice agenda that emerged from Catholic teaching. Liberation theology, liberation psychology (Watkins & Shulman, 2008), and other liberatory perspectives have promoted the goals of social justice in a global world, and worked to reframe the notion of development, which has become associated in very negative ways with patterns of exploitation and resource depletion, and practices of stigmatizing other nations as under-developed. Watkins and Shulman (2008) trace the history of liberation psychology as it evolved from liberation theology, including liberation theology's challenges to governing elites and colonizing interests in Latin America and its critique of development. Quoting Gustavo Gutiérrez, the Peruvian priest and founder of liberation theology, Watkins and Shulman (2008) shed light on the social justice goals of such movement, "Peace, justice, love and peace are not private realities; they are not only internal attitudes. They are social realities, implying a historical liberation (Gutiérrez, 1988, p. 167)" (Watkins & Shulman, 2008, p. 32).

According to Watkins and Shulman (2008), liberation theology and psychology have focused on understanding, supporting, and recognizing local interests, goals, dreams, and identities. The theorizing by the present authors in Chapter 2 about a Maternal Cosmos and the power of the symbolic order to disrupt dominant practices, while grounding and nurturing creativity, dreaming, generativity, love and dialogue, resonates deeply with Watkin's and Shulman's commentaries on the connections between theorizing and human relationships and praxis. The global project of social justice for all older persons must build on these liberation movements.

The profession of social work has a deep and rich tradition in social justice, as reflected in its NASW Code of Ethics (2017):

> ...The mission of the social work profession is rooted in a set of core values. These core values, embraced by social workers throughout the profession's history, are the foundation of social work's unique purpose and perspective:
>
> - service
> - social justice
> - dignity and worth of the person
> - importance of human relationships
> - integrity
> - competence.
>
> (Preamble, NASW Code of Ethics, 2017)

The following is an excerpt from a speech delivered on May 22, 2000, by Mary Ann Quaranta, social work educator who served as president of the National Association of Social Workers and Dean of the Fordham Graduate

School of Social Service for 25 years, in a 50-year retrospective of the social work profession:

> A great many changes occurred during these 50 years in our society, in our social structures, in our social mores ... There have been dramatic changes in social work and in social work education as well and these changes have been reflected in education, and we have made every effort to have our curriculum and our field practice as *au courant* as possible. The 50 years have brought increasing recognition to our profession as being a meaningful one and as improving life for others and we have developed a greater level of credibility in the academy for our research and for developing our own solid knowledge base. During the past decades, we have been licensed or certified for practice in all 50 states. Some things have really not changed, however. What has not changed is the fundamental theme of our profession, which is our mission to promote social justice in our society and in all communities where we work. Also, what has not changed is the unacceptable percentage of people in our society and in all societies around the world who are marginalized, who are destitute, who are forlorn, who are downtrodden and oppressed, and not experiencing the bare minimum requirement for a decent quality of life.
>
> (Quaranta, 2000, Fordham University Archives, unpublished speech)

As Quaranta expressed so well, the fundamental theme of social justice as a core value of social work has remained intact across the years and generations. This is a goal that has been embraced by many other professions and disciplines and should serve as a ground for interdisciplinary collaboration in the aging and health fields. A renewed commitment to older persons who are marginalized, destitute, and oppressed must be an urgent social justice goal of the next decades for psychology, social work, public health, and all the professions and disciplines involved in any way with aging and health work.

Professor Lawrence O. Gostin (2014) puts it this way:

> Although overall population health is vitally important, justice requires a significant reduction in health disparities between the well-off and the poor ... Global health with justice demands that society embed fairness into the environment in which people live and equitably allocate services, with particular attention to the needs of the most disadvantaged.
>
> (Gostin, 2014, pp. 412–413)

In advocating for a firm commitment to social justice goals, we envision policy change that would prioritize investments in education for all persons across the life course—investments that would give them a fair chance at a good life. The most compelling research on aging and health speaks to the impact of education on life expectancy, healthy life expectancy, and health and well being outcomes (Olshansky et al., 2012; Olshansky, 2015), such as reducing risks of serious illness. There is accumulating evidence to support this claim. A recent snapshot of older people with serious illness compiled by the Kaiser Family Foundation (2017) shows clearly the relationship between health and education: seriously ill older adults are much more likely than their older adult peers without serious illness to be female (75% versus 53%), widowed (42% versus 24%), earn an annual income of less than $40,000 (64% versus 38%), and have a high school education or less (71% versus 40%), and are somewhat more likely than their peers to be black (18% versus 9%) or Hispanic (12% versus 5%) (Kaiser Family Foundation, 2017). In another recently issued report by the *Lancet* Commission on Dementia Prevention, Intervention and Care (Livingston et al., 2017), the Commission describes education as a modifiable risk factor for dementia. The authors of the report state that low educational level is believed to result in vulnerability to cognitive decline on account of its impact on cognitive reserve. Cognitive reserve makes it possible for older persons to maintain function, even in the presence of brain pathology.

Foregrounding education across the lifespan—and across generations—is the bedrock of the public health approach and its essential concerns with advancing the goals of social justice for all members of society and will determine to a great extent the future of that society. A society that denies persons an education consigns them to a life of poverty and illness that continues into their later years.

C.   *Sustainable social solidarity: Social protection and universal health coverage*

From Gostin to Reinhardt to Gutiérrez, Watkins and Shulman and Jennings, we have a well-established cadre of scholars and advocates who espouse common principles of social justice and social solidarity. Social justice and social solidarity are mutually re-enforcing and interdependent frameworks and practices. These frameworks and practices are relevant to the UN's Sustainable Development Goals, specifically SDG 1–3, the implementation of nationally appropriate social protection systems, which include floors or defined essential levels of security as part of the main sustainable development goal to end poverty in all its forms everywhere. In a recent editorial on "Achieving sustainable solidarity development goals," (*Lancet*, 2017) The *Lancet* acknowledges that the meanings of social solidarity and social security vary. A focus on social protection as a goal that is essential to eradicating poverty is helpful in building both a national and global consensus around social solidarity and social justice.

The UN's International Labor Organization (ILO) Report on "World Social Protection" (2017) defines social protection or social security as a human right and inclusive of a set of policies and programs designed to reduce poverty and vulnerability across the lifespan. The Report highlights the state of social protection for older persons worldwide with respect to both pensions and universal health coverage:

- Worldwide, 68% of retirement-age people receive an old-age pension.
- Benefit levels are often low and not adequate to push older persons out of poverty, remaining a challenge in many countries.
- Pension and other benefit expenditures for older persons account for 6.9% of GDP on average, with large variations across regions.
- Fiscal consolidation or austerity pressures in many countries continue to jeopardize the long-term adequacy of pensions, reflecting a fragile balance between sustainability and adequacy in the context of ageing populations.
- Long-term care (LTC) is mostly needed by older persons with limited ability to care for themselves due to a range of conditions.
- Over 48% of the world's population live in countries which do not provide any LTC protection to older persons; women are disproportionately affected.
- Another 46.3% of the older global population are largely excluded from LTC, due to narrow means-testing regulations that require older persons to be poor in order to become eligible for LTC services.
- Only 5.6% of the global population live in countries that provide LTC coverage based on national legislation that covers the whole population.
- Given aging populations and demographics, LTC needs to be properly addressed by public policies.
- Globally, approximately 57 million unpaid "voluntary" workers are bridging the LTC workforce gap and carrying the burdens of this work, many of whom are women who provide informal care for family members. (World Social Protection Report 2017–2019, Executive Summary)

We strongly support the recommendations of the ILO for universal health coverage including long-term care for all older persons.

IV.   Conclusion

It presents a challenging task to write the conclusion for a book on a subject with as much gravitas as aging and public health, and one that encompasses such a vast breadth of concerns affecting older persons and the society as a whole. We choose to bring these discussions to a close with final reflections about possibility for older persons—possibility for agency, transcendence, and hope—in light of conditions of suffering we described. This is an imagining of a refashioned world order in which no one is left behind—not a type of transactional social contract, but rather a kind of social solidarity that is built on deep social and relational connections and on felt obligation to one another.

In Chapter 1, we discussed the framework of successful aging and the positive focus that characterizes such framework, but provided a counterpoint with an equally important approach-problematizing the experience of older persons. We have approached that problem-framing through the lens of social ecology and its ecosystems, including macro-level neoliberal ideologies. Such problem framing is a condition precedent to a meaningful policy process and to designing public health responses and solutions at the population level that will address older persons' unmet needs, as well as opportunities for their flourishing and well being.

In Chapter 2, we drew attention to the distinctions between immanence and transcendence and between the psychological and the transcendental, suggesting that the transcendental perspective may offer an opportunity for transcendence in the phenomenological sense that we described—in other words, in a way that permits both deeper understanding of the sense-making achievements of human subjectivity and a return to the world with that transcendentally informed knowledge. This is a response to Bruce Jennings's concern about the privatization of transcendence, or what we would describe as the neoliberal self's appropriation of the world. The transcendental perspective is neither attached to any region nor to any psychological subject. It exists prior to the world, and therefore is not amenable to being privatized. It occupies no position in the world but offers a point of access to the world prior to its being. We analogized this transcendental perspective or moment of consciousness to a re-symbolized and degenderized Maternal Cosmos that is a primordial, welcoming home and a ground of generativity and agency.

We also highlighted findings from studies of suffering among older adults (Morrissey, 2011, 2015) that suggest that in the midst of suffering, there is the abiding presence of Maternal dimensions of existence that are remembered and re-enacted, and afford opportunity for agency, resilience, generativity, and hope, even for those older persons who may face the most abject suffering or are nearing the end of life.

Finally, rejecting the theory that successful aging is entirely within the power of the individual, we call for radical changes in social policy that will modify conditions of health and well being, rebalance our global resources, and prioritize investments in social protection and social security, such as education for all persons, especially women and girls who are often lagging behind their male counterparts. We express confidence in the promise of palliative systems of care and public health strategies for translating integrated palliative care programs and services into the field—and echo the calls for *palliative care for all*, *palliative care everywhere*, and *palliative environments*. Such strategies offer the best chance for reducing widening disparities and assuring that every older person in the society has equitable access to health facilities, goods and services and their equitable distribution, and can participate meaningfully in communities of care and in co-constituting liberatory social practices.

References

Cubanski, J., Casillas, G., & Damico, A. (2015). *Poverty among seniors: An updated analysis of national and state level poverty rates under the official and supplemental poverty measures.* Menlo Park, CA: Henry J. Kaiser Family Foundation.

Gomez-Batiste, X. & Connor, Stephen. (Eds.). (2017). *Building integrated palliative care programs and services.* Catalonia, Spain: WHO Collaborating Centre Public Health Palliative Care Programmes.

Gostin, L. (2014). *Global health law.* Cambridge, MA: Harvard University Press.

Gostin, L. (2017, December). The "great" generation and a not-so-great health system. *Milbank Quarterly, 95.* Retrieved from: www.milbank.org/quarterly/articles/great-generation-not-great-health-system/.

Gutierrez, G. (1988) *A theology of liberation: History, politics and salvation.* (Trans. and Ed. Sr. C. Inda & J. Eagleson). Maryknoll, NY: Orbis Books.

Hall, S., Petkova, H., Tsouros, A.D., Costantini, M., & Higginson, I.J. (Eds.) (2011). *Palliative care for older people: Better practices.* Copenhagen, Denmark: WHO Regional Office for Europe.

International Labour Organization (ILO) (2017). *World Social Protection Report 2017–2019: Universal social protection to achieve the sustainable development goals.* Geneva, Switzerland: ILO.

Lynn, J. (2016). *MediCaring communities: Getting what we want and need in frail old age at an affordable cost.* Altarum Institute and Joanne Lynn.

Lancet. (2017). Achieving sustainable solidarity development goals. *Lancet, 390*(10113), 2605. Retrieved from: www.thelancet.com/journals/lancet/article/PIIS0140-6736(17)33303-2/fulltext.

Levinas, E. (1969). *Totality and infinity: An essay on exteriority.* Pittsburgh, PA: Duquesne University Press.

Levy, A. (2017, December 17 & 25). Ophelia Dahl's National Health Service. *New Yorker.* Retrieved from: www.newyorker.com/magazine/2017/12/18/ophelia-dahls-national-health-service.

Livingston, G., Sommerlad, A., Orgeta, V., Costafreda, S.G., Huntley, J., Ames, D., ... Ballard, C. (2017). Dementia prevention, intervention and care. *Lancet, 390*: 2673–2734.

Morrissey, M.B. (2011). *Suffering and decision making among seriously ill elderly women.* (Doctoral dissertation, Fordham University). Retrieved from: http://fordham.bepress.com/dissertations/AAI3458134/.

Morrissey, M.B. (2015). *Suffering narratives of older adults.* New York, NY: Routledge.

NASW Code of Ethics. (2017). Retrieved from: www.socialworkers.org/About/Ethics/Code-of-Ethics/Code-of-Ethics-English.

Olshansky, S.J. (2015). The demographic transformation of America. *Daedalus, the Journal of the American Academy of Arts & Sciences, 144*(2), 13–19.

Olshansky, S.J., Antonucci, T., Berkman, L., Binstock, R.H., Boersch-Supan, A., Cacioppo, J.T., ... Rowe, J. (2012). Differences in life expectancy due to race and educational differences are widening, and may not catch up. *Health Affairs, 31*(8), 1803–1813.

Quaranta, M.A. (2000). *Fifty-year retrospective of social work profession.* Fordham University Archives, Unpublished talk.

Reinhardt, U. (2012, June 29). Health care: Solidarity vs. rugged individualism. *New York Times*. Retrieved from: https://economix.blogs.nytimes.com/2012/06/29/health-care-solidarity-vs-rugged-individualism/.

Watkins, M., & Shulman, H. (2008). *Toward psychologies of liberation*. UK: Palgrave Macmillan.

Bibliography

Dijulio, B., Hamel, L., Wu, B., Brodie, M. (2017, November). *Serious illness in late life: The public's views and experiences*. Menlo Park, CA: Kaiser Family Foundation.

Jennings, B. (2016). *Ecological governance: Toward a new social contract with the Earth*. Morgantown: West Virginia University Press.

Appendix A: Caregiving resources

The Administration for Community Living (ACL) is a federal agency that supports programs that help support and empower those caring for older adults and people with disabilities.

- The National Family Caregiver Support Program (www.acl.gov/node /314) supports programs for family and informal caregivers.
- The Lifespan Respite Care Program (www.acl.gov/node/441) works to improve respite supports and services for caregivers of older adults and people with disabilities.

The National Alliance for Caregiving partners with other caregiving associations and groups to provide additional resources to help family caregivers cope with the challenges of caring for a loved one.

Caregiver Action Network
www.caregiveraction.org/
Provides resources from the Caregiver Action Network, including a peer forum, a story sharing platform, the family caregiver tool box.

Caring.com
www.caring.com
This resource is an online destination for family caregivers seeking information and support offering a comprehensive directory of eldercare services and advice from a team of leaders in geriatric medicine, law, finance, and housing.

Eldercare Locator
www.eldercare.gov/Eldercare.NET/Public/Index.aspx
This locator, a public service of the U.S. Administration on Aging, links those who need assistance with state and local area agencies on aging and community-based organizations that serve older adults and their caregivers.

Family Caregiver Alliance
http://caregiver.org/node/3831
The National Center on Caregiving (NCC) works in every state to advance cost-effective policies and programs for caregivers; it serves as a central source of information on caregiving and long-term care issues.

Financial Steps for Caregivers
WISER (Women's Institute for a Secure Retirement)
www.wiserwomen.org
This resource is designed to help identify financial decisions caregivers face to address short-term and long-term financial security, including retirement.

Kaiser Family Foundation
http://files.kff.org/attachment/Report-Serious-Illness-in-Late-Life-The -Publics-Views-and-Experiences
Serious Illness in Late Life: The Public's Views and Experiences (November 2017)

Lotsa Helping Hands
www.lotsahelpinghands.com
This is a free caregiving coordination web service that provides a private, group calendar where tasks for which a caregiver needs assistance can be posted. Family and friends may visit the site and sign up online for a task. The website generates a report showing who has volunteered for which tasks and which tasks remain unassigned. The site tracks each task and notification and reminder emails are sent to the appropriate parties.

National Family Caregiver Support Program
www.acl.gov/programs/support-caregivers/national-family-caregiver -support-program
This support program provides grants and funds a variety of supports that assist caregivers.

National Transitions of Care Coalition
www.NTOCC.org
NTOCC offers resources to help better understand transitional challenges and empower caregivers.

Next Step in Care
www.nextstepincare.org
This resource provides guides for planning transitions for chronically or seriously ill individuals, for caregivers, and health care providers.

U.S. Food and Drug Administration, Office of Women's Health
fda.gov/womeninclinicaltrials
FDA's Tips for Caregivers website provides tips for caregivers of older adults, young children, teens, and people with special needs.

Appendix B: Ecology of policy
Description of public policy making process

Public Policy Making

This appendix describes and gives examples of *public policy making*, that is, the authoritative decisions of the three branches of government—legislative, executive, or judicial, that are designed to influence others' actions, behaviors, or decisions (Longest, 2016).

> *Example of Executive Branch Policy Making*: U.S. Department of Health & Human Services Determination that a public health emergency exists nationwide as result of opioid crisis (October 2017). (See www.hhs.gov/sites /default/files/opioid%20PHE%20Declaration-no-sig.pdf)

Types of Public Policy Making

- Social Policy—Decisions of government addressing social problems
- Social Welfare Policy—Decisions of government concerning social provision and wealth redistribution
- Aging Policy—Decisions of government concerning older adults
- Health Policy—Decisions of government concerning attainment of health
- Public Health Policy—Decisions of government concerning the health of the public or populations, including health infrastructure and health systems
- Global Public Health Policy—Decisions of government concerning global health or the health of populations across the world, operationalization of the right to health and the right to the enjoyment of the highest attainable standard of physical and mental health. Global public health also includes the responsibilities of nation states and institutions of governance, such as the World Health Organization.

> *Example of Public Health Policy Making*: In its 2011 report, "The Public's Health: Revitalizing Law and Policy to Meet New Challenges," the Institute of Medicine (IOM) reframes good health as encompassing good medical care plus effective public policy. The IOM (2011) also enumerates categories of law and policy relating to public health:

1 *Laws establishing the structure, function, and authority of federal, state and local government public health agencies.*
2 *Statutes and other policies designed to achieve specific health objectives, for example, taxing tobacco products and requiring immunization for school entry.*
3 *Policies in other areas of government and intersectoral strategies that have health effects, such as education, transportation, land use planning, and agriculture.*

Below are essential public health functions and services:

- *Monitor health status to identify and solve community health problems*
- *Diagnose and investigate health problems and health hazards in the community*
- *Inform, educate, and empower people about health issues*
- *Mobilize community partnerships and actions to identify and solve health problems*
- *Develop policies and plans that support individual and community health efforts*
- *Enforce laws and regulations that protect health and ensure safety*
- *Link people to needed personal health services and assure the provision of health care when otherwise unavailable*
- *Assure a competent public and personal health care workforce*
- *Evaluate effectiveness, accessibility, and quality of personal and population-based health services*
- *Conduct research to gain new insights and guide development of innovative solutions to health problems*

(Birkhead, 2012; IOM, 2011; Public Health Functions Steering Committee, 1994. Retrieved from: www.cdc.gov/nphpsp/essentialservices.html)

Forms of policies

- Laws (federal, state, and local)
- Rules or regulations
- Implementation decisions or guidance
- Judicial decisions (federal or state courts) (Longest, 2016)

Example of Federal Law: Affordable Care Act (2010)
Example of Federal Regulation: Health Insurance Portability and Accountability Act or HIPAA (1996)
Example of Guidance: New York State Department of Health Palliative Care Law Guidance (see www.health.ny.gov/professionals/patients /patient_rights/palliative_care/)
Example of Judicial Decision of U.S. Supreme Court: Cruzan (1990)

Categories of policies

*   Allocative—Provide benefits to a particular group or class of individuals or oganizations

    Example: Affordable Care Act (2010) Subsidies (see www.valuepenguin .com/understanding-aca-subsidies)

*   Regulatory—Designed to assure policy objectives are met
    *   Market-entry restrictions
    *   Rate- or price-setting controls on health services providers
    *   Quality controls on provision of health services
    *   Market-preserving controls
    *   Social regulation

    Example: Centers for Medicare & Medicaid Services (CMS) Hospice Quality Reporting Program (Longest, 2016)

Phases of public policy making process

*   Policy formulation
    *   Agenda setting
        *   Problem framing
        *   Situational analysis
        *   Political contexts
        *   Possible solutions or policy alternatives
    *   Development of legislation
        *   Initiating and drafting legislative proposals
        *   Legislative committee and subcommittee review and approval process
        *   Budget process

    Example: Older Americans Act (see https://legcounsel.house.gov /Comps/Older%20Americans%20Act%20Of%201965.pdf)

*   Policy implementation
    *   Design
    *   Rulemaking
    *   Operating
    *   Evaluating
*   Policy modification
    *   Applicable to all phases

    Example: Older Americans Reauthorization Act of 2016 (see www .congress.gov/bill/114th-congress/senate-bill/192)

- Policy impact assessment (see program evaluation)

  Example: Health Impact Assessment (Longest, 2016)

  Example of Public Policy Making Process: Public Health Strategy for Palliative Care
  - Policy development
  - Access to essential medicines
  - Education and training
  - Policy implementation (Stjernswärd, Foley, & Ferris, 2007)

Types of Program Evaluations

- Process evaluation
  - Formative
- Outcome evaluation
  - Summative
- Cost-benefit
- Cost-effectiveness (Longest, 2016)

  Example: The IOM identifies evaluation (IOM, 2011) as a critical public health tool in assessing the impact of laws and policies, and as an essential public health function and service: *Evaluate effectiveness, accessibility, and quality of personal and population-based health services.*

Policy Analysis

An approach to solving social problems involving systematic comparison and evaluation of evidence and alternatives by public actors (Weimer & Vining, 2005).

- Four-Pronged Policy Analysis Framework
  - Who are beneficiaries? Allocation; selective to universal criteria; operationalizing eligibility. *Example*: Older adults
  - What is benefit? Provision, cash, in-kind, other. *Example*: Medicare Hospice Benefit
  - What is financing? Public/private/mixed; types of taxes. *Example:* Medicare program
  - What is delivery system? Public/private/mixed; centralization or decentralization. *Example:* Medicare approved hospice program (Gilbert & Terrell, 2013)
- Bardach's Eight-Step Approach
  - Frame problem
  - Collect evidence
  - Identify alternatives

- Select criteria
- Project outcomes
- Evaluate trade-offs
- Make decision
- Report on decision and decision process (Bardach, 2005)
- Evaluation Criteria for Value-Critical Social Policies and Programs Analysis
  - Equity
  - Adequacy
  - Efficiency (Chambers & Wedel, 2005; Stone, 2002)

Policy practice and advocacy

Policy practice seeks to change policies in legislative, agency, and community settings. The aim of *policy advocacy* is to change social policies for the benefit of powerless or vulnerable groups (Jansson, 2008).

> *Examples of National and Regional Advocacy Organizations*: American Heart Association, American Planning Association, American Psychological Association, American Public Health Association, American Society on Aging, Gerontological Society of America, National Hospice and Palliative Care Organization, Collaborative for Palliative Care, New York

Policy competence

Competence is a set of skills or knowledge, either basic or specialized knowledge or expertise, in a particular area of policy or policy practice. Four skills of policy practitioners are: political competencies, analytic competencies, interactional competencies, and value-clarifying competencies (Jansson, 2008).

Workforce education and training and public education

- Professional Education and Training Goals and Content Areas
  - Policy competence
  - Clinical competence
    - Clinical knowledge and skills
    - Interpersonal communication and conflict negotiation skills
    - Knowledge in ethics, ethics committees, and ethical decision making
    - Organizational and systems knowledge
  - Building professional capacities
  - Affording professional development and interprofessional, cross-sectoral collaboration opportunities

- Public Education across the Lifespan for Targeted Groups
  - School-age children and high school and college students
  - Medical and other graduate students
  - Non-elderly adults
  - Persons with chronic or serious illness
  - Family caregivers
  - Health care agents
  - Surrogates
  - Communities and community leaders
  - Judges

References

Bardach, E. (2005). *A practical guide for policy analysis. The eightfold path to more effective problem solving.* Washington, DC: CQ Press.

Birkhead, G. (2012). Overview: Assuring the public's health: What is "public health" and what is the role of the law? *New York State Bar Association Health Law Journal, 17*(2), 26–31.

Chambers, D.E., & Wedel, K.R. (2005). *Social policy and social programs.* Boston, MA: Pearson Education.

Gilbert, N., & Terrell, P. (2013). *Dimensions of social welfare policy.* Boston, MA: Pearson.

Institute of Medicine (IOM). (2011). *The public's health: Revitalizing law and policy to meet new challenges.* Washington, DC: National Academies Press. https://doi.org/10.17226/13093

Jansson, B.S. (2008). *Becoming an effective policy advocate. From policy practice to social justice.* Belmont, CA: Thomson Brooks Cole.

Longest, B.B. (2016). *Health policy making in the United States.* Chicago, IL: Health Administration Press.

Public Health Functions Steering Committee. (1994). *The public health workforce: An agenda for the 21st century. Full report of the public health functions project.* Washington, DC: Department of Health & Human Services.

Stjernswärd, J., Foley, K.M., & Ferris, F.D. (2007). The public health strategy for palliative care. *Journal of Pain and Symptom Management, 33*(5), 486–493.

Stone, D. (2002). *Policy paradox: The art of political decision making.* New York and London: Norton & Company.

Weimer, D.L., & Vining, A.R. (2005). *Policy analysis: Concepts and practice.* Upper Saddle River, NJ: Pearson.

Appendix C: Psychosocial support

Psychosocial care addresses the psychological, emotional, and social well being of patients and family members. Psychosocial needs should be regularly assessed to identify emotional distress, areas of concern for appropriate interventions, and referrals. Assessment and interventions in psychological, psychiatric, and social care help individuals and family members cope with the challenges associated with advanced illness.

Many people describe a variety of concerns after they receive a diagnosis of advanced illness that may include, but are not limited to:

- Experiencing depression and/or anxiety
- Maintaining their independence or sense of control
- Making treatment decisions
- Communicating effectively with the medical team
- Navigating the medical system
- Discussing diagnosis and prognosis with children, family, and friends
- Handling the financial strain of illness

Communication

Communication is critical for high-quality care. Using empathy, compassion, and listening skills are key components of effective communication. Communication can include several factors covering the illness trajectory that integrate individuals and their families and/or caregivers.

Key components include:

- Discussions regarding diagnosis or prognosis, and communication of risks
- Information gathering and exploration of physical, psychosocial, and existential/spiritual needs, and of preferences/wishes
- Providing advice, discussing complex decisions, sharing decision making and goals of care, and discussions incorporating advance care planning
- Relationship building and responding to difficult emotions

Psychological and Emotional Care

Patients and family members face a range of issues when facing illness. Understanding the individual's strengths and coping styles, along with values and goals, is critical. If psychological distress is identified, the appropriate types of support should be offered and encouraged. Depression, anxiety, or overwhelming sadness can be addressed to improve the remaining quality of life. Individuals approach challenges in life with a wide range of responses, which are linked to their psychological strengths and vulnerabilities.

Emotional suffering is common among patients adjusting to advanced and chronic conditions; psychological distress is natural when an individual is confronted with the knowledge of prolonged illness and end-of-life issues. Anxiety and fears about what the future holds can adversely affect treatment compliance and quality of life. Psychological distress can vary during disease progression; the individual's coping strategies can play a significant role in adjusting to the challenges the illness presents.

Assessment

To alleviate psychological distress, it is recommended that assessments of psychological support needs are provided throughout the disease trajectory. Levels of psychological distress should be assessed with a screening/diagnostic instrument.

Intervention

The appropriate psychological intervention will depend on the level of psychological distress, previous history with psychological problems, the availability of social support, and disease prognosis. Psychological support requires listening to the individual's worries and emotional distress, normalizing reactions, and offering supportive communication. Alleviating distress can involve psychological techniques to facilitate coping and problem solving. Individuals with advanced illness are at greater risk of psychological distress; professionals must recognize common manifestations of distress, and offer psychological and psychiatric interventions when appropriate. Depression and anxiety may be treated with pharmacotherapy, counseling and psychotherapy, and complementary therapies. There are various models of counseling that can be offered individually or within groups.

Counseling

Before initiating counseling, a clinical assessment should be completed that includes psychosocial history and exploration of the cause of distress. Delivery of counseling, including the frequency, duration of sessions, location, and format of treatment, should be flexible and mindful of the stage of illness and medical status. Whatever approach is taken, it should be tailored to the specific needs and preferences of the patient and family.

Social Support

Comprehensive assessment of social support needs is critical in person-centered models. It is critical to understand the individual in the context of his/her family and social network (e.g., roles within the family and social capital), especially as the illness progresses. For those no longer able to financially support themselves and their families, referrals to sources of funding and support should be explored.

Bibliography

Gómez-Batiste, X., & Connor, S. (2017). *Building integrated palliative care programs and services.* Catalonia, Spain: Liberduplex.

Institute of Medicine (IOM). (2008). *Cancer care for the whole patient: Meeting psychosocial health needs.* Washington, DC: National Academies Press.

Appendix D: Resources and program examples for older adults

Federal Resources

U.S. Department of Health & Human Services (HHS) (https://www.hhs.gov) has multiple agencies that provide programs that improve the well being of older adults. Programs for seniors and resources include:

> NIHSeniorHealth (www.nia.nih.gov/health) (National Institute on Aging, National Institutes of Health)
> Health and wellness information for older adults.
>
> Senior Health (http://www.healthfinder.gov/scripts/SearchContext .asp?topic=1187)(Healthfinder.gov)
> Information about health for older adults.
>
> Senior Health en Español (http://www.healthfinder.gov/scripts /SearchContext.asp?topic=1187&Branch=5&lang=2&doclang=2) (Healthfinder.gov)
> Spanish-language health information.
>
> Eldercare Locator (https://eldercare.acl.gov/Public/Index.aspx) (Administration on Aging)
> Connects services for older adults and their families.
>
> Administration on Aging (www.aoa.acl.gov/) (Administration for Community Living)

Information about services and programs designed to help older adults live independently in their homes and communities. The aging and disability networks are made up of local, state, and national organizations that work to support older adults and people with disabilities. While there are many similarities in the services and supports that are offered for older adults that aim to keep them healthy and independent, the missions of the networks vary.

Administration for Community Living supports these networks; their website has a comprehensive list of programs and services, here are general categories:

- Aging and Disability Resource Centers (www.acl.gov/node/699)—These centers provide information and counseling about long-term services and supports.
- Americans with Disabilities Act National Network (www.acl.gov/node/409)—Regional centers provide information, training, and technical assistance to individuals, businesses, and agencies.
- Area Agencies on Aging (www.acl.gov/node/593)—These agencies address the needs of older adults at the regional and local level through services and supports (e.g., home-delivered meals and homemaker assistance) to support independent living.
- Assistive Technology (www.acl.gov/node/411)—These programs support making assistive technology devices and services more available and accessible to individuals with disabilities and their families.
- Centers for Independent Living (www.acl.gov/node/410)—These centers provide tools, resources, and supports for integrating people with disabilities fully into their communities.
- Protection and Advocacy Systems (www.acl.gov/node/70)—These state systems work to protect and empower individuals with disabilities and advocate on their behalf.
- Senior Centers and Supportive Services for Older Adults (www.acl.gov/node/311)—This program funds senior centers that coordinate services for older adults, such as congregate meals, community education, health screening, exercise and health promotion programs, and transportation.
- State Councils on Developmental Disabilities (www.acl.gov/node/467)—These organizations identify and address the most pressing needs of people with developmental disabilities to promote self-determination, integration, and inclusion.
- State Units on Aging (www.acl.gov/node/592)—These state-level agencies develop and administer plans to provide assistance for older adults, families.

Examples of aging in place and community resources

Village to Village Network is national organization that enables community members to create aging in place models called "Villages." Villages work to create services and supports that help older adults remain in their homes. A full list of local villages throughout the Unites States can be found at the Village to Village website at www.vtvnetwork.org.

AARP Livable Communities supports the efforts in local and regional areas to provide age-friendly communities, including housing and transportation, a range of services for residents of all ages to participate in community life. For a list of which towns and cities are in the AARP Network: www.aarp.org /livable-communities/.

Resources for individuals with cancer and their family members

Gilda's Club and Cancer Support Community make up the largest professionally led nonprofit network of cancer support worldwide, offer the highest quality social and emotional support for people impacted by cancer, and their family members. To find a local Gilda's Club or Cancer Support Community, www.cancersupportcommunity.org/FindLocation.

Appendix E: Elder Abuse, Maltreatment, and Neglect Resources

Administration for Community Living, Protecting Rights
and Preventing Abuse
www.acl.gov/programs/protecting-rights-and-preventing-abuse

Benjamin Rose Institute on Aging
http://benrose.org

Brookdale Center for Healthy Aging, Hunter College, CUNY
https://brookdale.org

Centers for Disease Control and Prevention (CDC) Elder Abuse
Definitions
www.cdc.gov/violenceprevention/elderabuse/definitions.html

Consumer Financial Protection Bureau (CFPB)
www.consumerfinance.gov/practitioner-resources/resources-for
-older-adults/

Elder Justice Coalition (EJC)
http://elderjusticecoalition.com

Elder Justice Coordinating Council (EJCC)
www.acl.gov/node/9

Elder Justice Initiative (EJI)
www.justice.gov/elderjustice

Eldercare Locator
www.eldercare.gov

Finger Lakes Geriatric Education Center (FLGEC)
www.urmc.rochester.edu/medicine/geriatrics/flgec.aspx

Institute on Violence, Abuse, and Trauma (IVAT)
www.ivatcenters.org

Long-Term Care Ombudsman Program
www.acl.gov/programs/protecting-rights-and-preventing-abuse
/long-term-care-ombudsman-program

National Adult Protective Services Association (NAPSA)
www.napsa-now.org

National Center on Elder Abuse (NCEA)
https://ncea.acl.gov

National Domestic Violence Hotline
www.thehotline.org/get-help

National Institute on Aging (NIA)
www.nia.nih.gov/health/elder-abuse

Office for Victims of Crime (OVC), Office of Justice, US Department of
Justice, Polyvictimization Curricula
www.ovcttac.gov/views/TrainingMaterials/dspOnline_polyvictimization
.cfm

Terra Nova Films, Elder Abuse Category
http://terranova.org/film-catalog/category/elder-abuse/

U.S. Department of Justice
elder.justice@usdoj.gov
www.justice.gov/elderjustice

Appendix F: Finger Lakes Geriatric Education Center—Geriatrics Workforce Enhancement Program

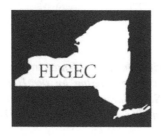

Purpose: The Finger Lakes Geriatric Education Center's goal is to develop a competent health care workforce that maximizes patient and family engagement and improves health outcomes for older adults by integrating geriatrics with primary care and creating linkages with community-based supports and services.

Education Center Highlights
- Support interprofessional, team-based, patient-centered health care for older adults
- Integrate geriatrics into evolving primary care delivery systems to provide coordinated and comprehensive health care
- Conduct outreach and education for patients, families, and caregivers to improve the health of older adults
- Develop distance-learning (online and teleconference) education and support for clinicians
- Target outreach to health care providers practicing in rural areas of upstate New York
- Special area of emphasis on education and training for health care professionals and caregivers related to Alzheimer's disease and other dementias

Geographic Area: As the map shows, the FLGEC concentrates its efforts in a well-defined 17 county area of the Finger Lakes region of New York State and serves primarily rural communities and the greater metropolitan region of Rochester, New York.

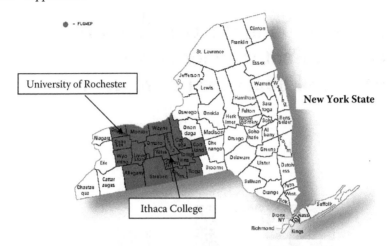

Funding: *The Finger Lakes Geriatric Education Center at the University of Rochester is made possible through grant funding by the Health Resources and Services Administration (HRSA) Bureau of Health Workforce under the Geriatric Workforce Enhancement Program (Grant # U1QHP28738)*

Strategic Collaborations and Partners:

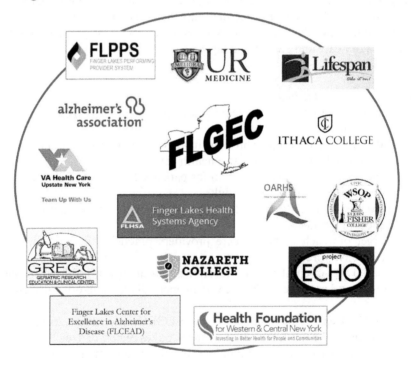

Caregiver Resources and Support
http://www.lifespan-roch.org/

Support and Education for Alzheimer's disease and related dementias
http://www.alz.org/rochesterny/

Rural Health Training
http://www.ithaca.edu/gerontology/

Education Center Collaborative Learning Environment®

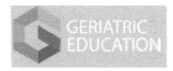 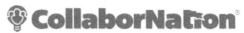

The Education Center Collaborative Learning Environment® is an online forum (distance learning) focused on the care of Older Adults which is offered free of charge for health care professionals through CollaborNation®.
Access the website: https://collabornation.net/login/geriatriceducation

Available Training Modules
- Geriatric Assessment
- Elder Abuse Prevention
- Chiropractic Care for Older Adults
- Geriatric Oncology
- Suicide in Older Adults
- Aging with Developmental and Intellectual Disabilities
- The 3Ds: Depression, Dementia, and Delirium
- Pain Self-Management
- Principles of Geriatric Pharmacotherapy
- Mindfulness

Project ECHO® in Geriatric Mental Health and Palliative Care

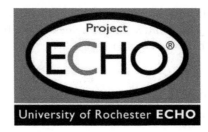

The Extension for Community Healthcare Outcomes (ECHO®) is an innovative model to improve access to complex chronic disease and specialty care in underserved communities through the use of videoconferencing technology. By providing community-based clinicians with skills and knowledge to treat complex patients in their own practices, ECHO® aims to improve health outcomes while also reducing the cost of care through a multidisciplinary team-based approach. **Access the Website: https://www.urmc.rochester.edu/project-echo.aspx.**

The Project ECHO®
- Supports the delivery of care by primary care practices and long-term care facility health care teams, especially in underserved and rural areas of New York State (NYS)
- Enhances expert care for older adults with dementia, mental health disorders, and palliative care
- Uses Technology (multipoint videoconferencing and Internet) to connect in team-based care
- Focuses on a Disease Management Model to reduce variation in processes of care and sharing "best practices" in a case-based learning format for the co-management of patients
- HIPAA-compliant web-based database to monitor outcomes

Finger Lakes Geriatric Education Center Staff
Project Director/PI: Thomas V. Caprio, MD, MPH, MSHPE
Project Co-Director/Senior Advisor: Jurgis Karuza, PhD
Project Coordinator: Laura Robinson, MPH
Director of Faculty Development: Annette Medina-Walpole, MD
Director of Quality Improvement: Suzanne Gillespie, MD
Director of Community Engagement & Planning Tobie Olsan, PhD, MPA, RN, CNL, NEA-BC, FNAP
Director of Caregiver Programs and Supports: Ann Marie Cook, MPA (Lifespan)
Director of Dementia Programs and Supports: Carol Podgorski, PhD, MPH, MS
Director of ECHO Programs: Michael Hasselberg, PhD, RN, PMHNP-BC
Director of Rural Outreach: Rohda Meador, PhD (Ithaca College)
External Advisory Committee Chair: Yeates Conwell, MD (Office for Aging Research & Health Services)

Contact Us
Thomas V. Caprio, MD
Director, Finger Lakes Geriatric Education Center
Phone: (585) 760-6364
Fax: (585) 760-6376
Email: Thomas_Caprio@urmc.rochester.edu

Laura Robinson, MPH
Project Coordinator, Finger Lakes Geriatric Education Center
Phone: (585) 760-6380
Fax: (585) 760-6376
Email: LauraM_Robinson@urmc.rochester.edu

Mailing Address
Finger Lakes Geriatric Education Center
University of Rochester School of Medicine and Dentistry
Department of Medicine, Division of Geriatrics and Aging
435 East Henrietta Road
Rochester, NY 14620

FLGEC Website: https://www.urmc.rochester.edu/medicine/geriatrics
/flgec.aspx

Appendix G: Photographs of Eduardo

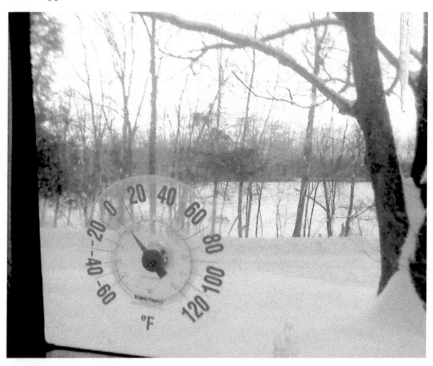

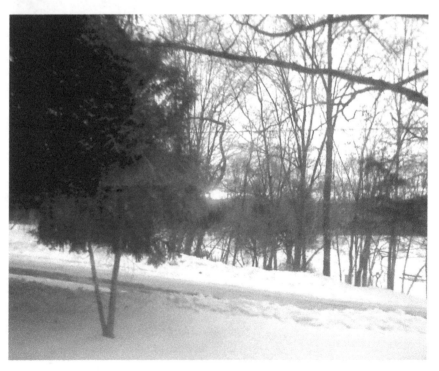

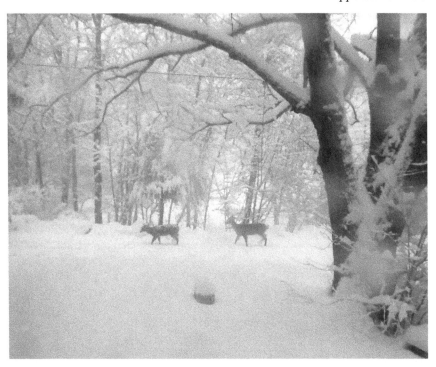

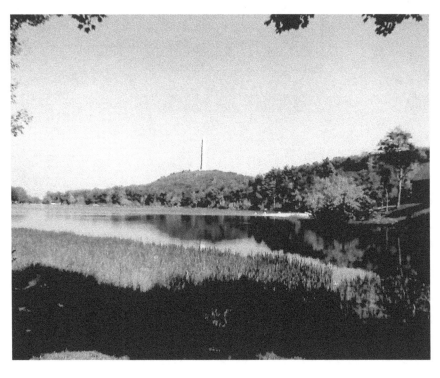

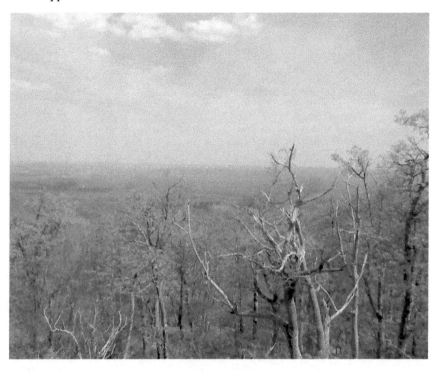

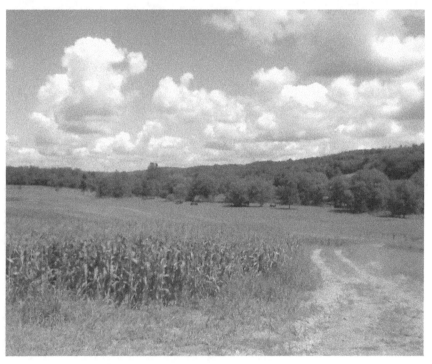

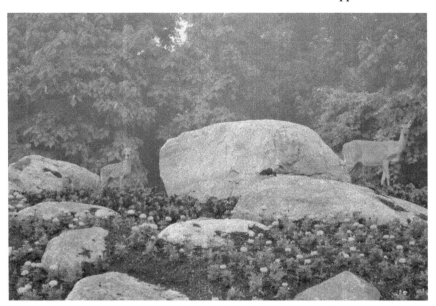

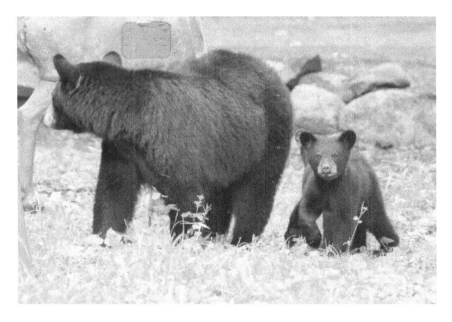

Index

Milton Keynes UK
Ingram Content Group UK Ltd.
UKHW040107071024
449327UK00019B/888